Peak Conditioning Training For Young Athletes

Strength and Fitness Programs Specifically Designed for 8- to 17-Year-Old Athletes

Thomas Emma

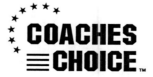

COACHES CHOICE™

ISBN: 1-58518-944-8
Library of Congress Control Number: 2005930484
Cover design: Jeanne Hamilton
Book layout: Jeanne Hamilton
Front cover photo: Dennis Dal Covey/Covey Media
Illustrations: Judy Picone-Fadeyev

Coaches Choice
P.O. Box 1828
Monterey, CA 93942
www.coacheschoice.com

Dedication

For Jack

Acknowledgments

I would first like to thank the editors and staff at Coaches Choice, especially Kristi Huelsing and Weiss Lancaster for their effort and skill in the book's production and marketing processes, respectively.

Special thanks to Judy Picone-Fadeyev, creative director of the Davinci Corporation, for her skill and timeliness with the illustrations. Thanks also to Michael Forrai of Minute Man Press for his work with the manuscript and for his computer expertise.

And finally, thanks to all the dedicated young athletes, especially those I work with regularly, who aspire on a daily basis to be the best they can be at their chosen sport(s).

Contents

Introduction

To say that youth sports are popular is perhaps the ultimate understatement. In fact, more children are participating in organized sports than ever before in our nation's history. This participation is broad based, including both boys and girls and encompassing the full spectrum of sports and programs. If recent years are any indication, the growth will continue to accelerate far into the future with no end in sight.

Unfortunately, while participation is very high in youth sports, physical preparation is alarmingly low. Very few young athletes prepare their bodies properly for the rigors of sports competition. The lack of preconditioning is cause for great concern, especially when you consider that many youngsters are multi-sport athletes who are competing throughout the year with very little downtime. This ultra-busy sports calendar leaves them vulnerable to injury, lackluster performance, and burnout.

Many believe the absence of preparation among young athletes is due to laziness and/or lack of time, which is not necessarily the case. The main culprit is instead the dearth of reliable information available relating to youth strength and conditioning. The overwhelming majority of books, videos, and periodicals dedicated to fitness and exercise are geared toward the adult population, either the general public or elite athletes. Youngsters are, for the most part, neglected. Without an age-appropriate format to follow, many improvement conscious young athletes find themselves either not training at all outside of their sport(s) or trying in vain to follow workout regimens designed for adults, or worse yet, for professional athletes.

Peak Conditioning Training for Young Athletes was created to fill this void. It will give youngsters and those who guide them (such as coaches, trainers, youth program directors, and parents) a comprehensive, easy-to-follow blueprint for youth strength and conditioning success. The book was carefully designed so that it can be incorporated by all young athletes regardless of age, physical maturity, athletic ability, or sport. In short, *Peak Conditioning Training for Young Athletes* offers something for everyone involved in youth sports—from the first year soccer player to the highly recruited high school basketball or football superstar.

The book itself begins with a thorough explanation of the three phases of a young athlete's development: acclamation, foundation, and maturation. Chapter 1 is the cornerstone of the book, and it will be necessary to refer to its contents regularly. As such, it must be read and understood prior to moving on to all other chapters—regardless of individual conditioning interests or sport-specific goals.

Chapters 2 through 4 focus on strategies for maintaining peak performance levels on a year-round basis—a key component considering the hectic sports schedules most young athletes adhere to in this day and age. Topics include warm-up, cool-down, flexibility, pre-movement training, recuperation, sleep, attitude, injuries, and youth sports nutrition.

Next up is a chapter on youth sports conditioning. Chapter 5 sets forth an organized program for improving cardiovascular efficiency in youngsters. It gives a detailed explanation of the body's energy systems, discusses the parameters of aerobic and anaerobic conditioning as they pertain to young athletes, and includes a variety of youth-appropriate exercise options and phase-specific conditioning training protocols.

Chapters 6, 7, and 8 expose the reader to the all-important and often controversial subject of youth strength training. Comprehensive coverage begins with the basics and principles of youth strength training (Chapter 6). Chapter 7 follows with more than 50 youth appropriate strength training exercises, complete with corresponding illustrations, explanations, and training tips. Chapter 8 concludes the section with phase-based strength training programs and workouts that will ensure that youngsters of all ages and ability levels get the most out of their strength training regimes.

Chapters 9 through 12 deal exclusively with movement and athleticism training. Among the topics discussed include balance (Chapter 9), speed (Chapter 10), quickness/agility (Chapter 11), and plyometrics (Chapter 12). Chapter 13 completes the book by providing a variety of cross training options that will help keep youngsters' workouts interesting and progressive.

Fusing the training programs and information contained in *Peak Conditioning Training for Young Athletes* with energy, determination, and hard work will prove to be an unbeatable, performance-enhancing combination—one that will allow youngsters to reach their full athletic potential, which is (after all) what it's all about for dedicated young athletes. I wish you the best of luck.

A Special Note to Readers

The exercises and drills explained and illustrated in this book follow carefully planned guidelines. By using this information as presented, you will experience the best possible results. As with all youth exercise programs, participants should see their physician before they begin.

1

Phases of a Young Athlete's Development

Research has shown that youngsters who strengthen and condition their bodies fully and properly will incur injury less frequently, perform better in their chosen sport(s), and gain more enjoyment and satisfaction from athletic activities. Those young people who work out regularly also tend to be more conscientious about their diet, abstain from drugs and alcohol, maintain a stable body weight, and generally feel better about themselves as individuals.

Notwithstanding these positive byproducts, it must be clearly understood that when it comes to physical training, children are not simply smaller versions of adults. They are not capable of engaging in workout regimes designed for full-grown individuals or those used by elite athletes. Youngsters have very unique fitness needs. As such, precautions must be taken, and age- and maturity-appropriate training protocols implemented for safe and productive results.

In this chapter, the training priorities for the three phases of a young athlete's development are discussed in detail, followed by 10 basic components everyone involved in youth physical training should be familiar with.

Phase 1: Acclamation — Seven to Ten Years Old

The number one priority of a fitness/exercise program for seven- through ten-year-olds is fun. Unless the program is enjoyable, young children will lose interest quickly and, in turn, all the other advantages of training will fall by the wayside. A non-competitive atmosphere should also be created, allowing youngsters to progress at their own pace without the pressure of comparison with other children.

From an athletic standpoint, the emphasis will be on mastering basic movement patterns, improving coordination, and learning proper running form and stretching techniques. Strength training will be slowly introduced in Phase 1, with the focus on high-repetition body weight, elastic band, and dumbbell exercises. Explosiveness training techniques such as plyometrics should be undertaken carefully with this age group. The stress on muscles, joints, and bones from high-impact training methods leaves pre-adolescent youngsters susceptible to injury. Adults supervising Phase 1 training programs will have to make determinations as to which youngsters have the strength and athletic ability to tolerate explosiveness training. Aerobic training is appropriate but should not be overdone, especially in the form of long-distance running, which can create problems for underdeveloped knees, shins, ankles, and feet. Specializing in a single sport or activity is also strongly discouraged at this stage of development.

Phase 1 conditioning workouts will be relatively brief (30 to 35 minutes or so) and reasonably fast paced. However, because young children's anaerobic systems are not fully developed, intensity levels must be carefully monitored so as to avoid overexertion. Attention spans are low at these ages, so sitting still is not an option for these little bundles of energy. Keeping everyone moving will help concentration levels remain as high as possible. Group activities such as relay races, circuit strength training, and partner-related drills usually work best. The liberal use of fitness props such as speed ladders, cones, and light medicine balls is also suggested to keep this group engaged.

Phase 2: Foundation — 11 to 13 Years Old

While fun and enjoyment is still a high priority in Phase 2, more attention will begin to be put on athletic development and improving sports performance. A congenial, supportive atmosphere will continue to be engendered during workouts; however, aspects of competition should be introduced at this time.

The biggest difference between Phase 1 and Phase 2 is that of training intensity. Because their anaerobic systems and musculatures are quickly developing, youngsters ages 11, 12, and 13 can tolerate much more physical stress than can their younger counterparts. Therefore, workouts will be more demanding and intense. The duration of the conditioning sessions will also increase to about 45 minutes or so for most children in this age range.

Strength training will take on a more prominent role in Phase 2. The concentration should be on exercising the core of the body (hips, lower back, and abdominal regions) and building a base of overall strength. More complicated movement patterns will also be presented during this phase, with the emphasis on changing direction and performing drills at higher rates of speed. Keep in mind that some children at the upper end of this age range may experience dynamic spurts in growth. As such, additional basic coordination and footwork drills should be continued from Phase 1 to help these youngsters deal with their ever-growing bodies. Aerobic capacity should continue to be developed through a variety of modalities (running, swimming, biking, etc.). Explosiveness training can be more aggressively prescribed during this stage of development as well. However, because youngsters at these ages are still susceptible to impact-related injuries, most will engage in simple plyometric drills such as tuck jumps, bounds, and barrier hops. To reduce the stress on the lower body, all explosiveness workouts should be performed on soft, even surfaces (rubberized running tracks, low-cut grass, semi-soft sand, etc.).

The ultimate goal of Phase 2, as the title of the section suggests, is to develop a foundation of strength, power, endurance, and athleticism for future athletic pursuits, which will become much more competitive and intense in the years to come. The better prepared Phase 2 youngsters are from a physical standpoint to deal with these new athletic challenges, the more success they will ultimately enjoy in later years.

Phase 3: Maturation — 14 to 17 Years Old

Training intensity and volume will be ramped up considerably in Phase 3. The majority of exercise sessions will be rigorous and, in many cases, span an hour or more. Workouts will continue to be relatively balanced and well rounded, especially during the off-season months. However, sport, need, and position-specific training protocols should now begin to be incorporated. For instance, a 15-year-old football lineman will spend more time strength training in the weight room than he will jogging around the running track. Similarly, late high school age volleyball and basketball players are best served using large portions of their workout hours performing drills designed to enhance jumping ability and explosiveness.

A variety of advanced training methods will be taught and incorporated for the first time in Phase 3, including ballistic stretching, combination barbell strength exercises, and intense explosiveness movements such as box jumps and dynamic medicine ball throws. Because of increases in physical stature, most Phase 3 youngsters will now be able to incorporate a full complement of exercise machines into their workouts. Both aerobic and anaerobic workouts will increase in duration and intensity in this phase as well.

Overtraining can become a common problem during Phase 3, as the introduction of advanced training techniques (combined with youngsters' ever-increasing tolerance for exercise) leads many athletes in this age range to overdo it. It is extremely important that coaches, trainers, and parents monitor youngsters' activity levels and remain ever-vigilant in recognizing the signs of overtraining, which may include losses in strength and power, lack of enthusiasm for workouts, and insomnia. Once overtraining is recognized, workouts should be scaled back immediately and accordingly. (Overtraining is discussed in more detail later in the chapter.)

Taking personal responsibility for athletic progress is a big part of Phase 3. While youngsters in Phases 1 and 2 will focus on following directions and learning proper workout protocol, athletes at this stage are encouraged to tune into their bodies and begin to develop an intuitive feel for which training strategies work best. Every youngster responds somewhat differently to workout stimulus. Therefore, finding the training methods that are most effective will save much time and energy—not to mention frustration—during the journey toward optimal physical condition. In fact, developing "training intuition" is as important a factor in achieving long-term athletic success as doing good old-fashioned hard work.

10 Basic Components of Youth Strength and Conditioning

1. Not All Youngsters Mature at the Same Rate

It is important to note that children of the same chronological age may be very different in terms of physical maturity. Some youngsters mature early and are able to make substantial gains in strength and speed at young ages. Others mature late and need time and patience to improve from a physical standpoint. The majority are somewhere in-between.

Of the three groups previously mentioned, late-maturing youngsters are of particular concern. The psychological burden of developing later than their peers can be a heavy one. However, this cloud of late maturation has a silver lining. Often the "late bloomers" turn out to be better, more successful athletes in the long haul than their early-developing counterparts. For confirmation, look no further than basketball all-time greats Michael Jordan, Julius Erving, and Scottie Pippen. All three of these superstars developed late physically and, because of lack of size and strength, were forced to perfect basketball skills, footwork, and coordination in order to compete during their formative years. Thus, when their physical attributes caught up with their skills and savvy, a state-of-the-art athlete emerged.

Adults involved with late developers should encourage them to take heart and not get discouraged. Let them know that their time will come. And if they don't believe it, make sure they're aware of the backgrounds of the previously mentioned basketball hall-of-famers.

2. Training for Youngsters Should Be Fun, Creative, and Interesting

Physical exercise is often associated with drudgery, a necessary evil in the quest toward reaching one's conditioning goals. While the majority of adults have a variety of reasons for working out (health benefits, cosmetic improvements, and social interaction to name a few), and can therefore tolerate a reasonable amount of tediousness from their fitness regimes, this is not the case for youngsters—especially children under 12 years of age. Young athletes require that all workouts be fun and enjoyable or their interest and performance will wane in short order. Once interest is lost, youngsters (as we all know) are quick to move on to the next activity, which will most likely have nothing whatsoever to do with keeping their bodies in shape.

It is up to those who devise and supervise youth fitness programs to create a fun and interesting training environment. Employing a variety of training strategies and remaining aware of how youngsters are responding to different modes of exercise are among the best ways to achieve this end. No stone should be left unturned. Be as creative as possible, and if something isn't working, don't hesitate to scrap it and move on to another drill, exercise, or activity. Incorporate teamwork, goal setting, and positive reinforcement to keep youngsters engaged and excited during workouts. With the right planning and attention, achieving top shape can be a fun, pleasurable experience—one to which youngsters look forward and on which they thrive.

3. The Long-Term Approach is Best

We've all heard the story of the race between the tortoise and the hare where the hare sprints out to a big lead at the start of the contest only to be caught and eventually passed and beaten by the slow, but consistent-moving, giant land tortoise. Young athletes, and those who guide them, can learn a lot from this popular fable.

When it comes to physical training, and most other things in life for that matter, the consistent, long-term approach usually wins out in the end. Young athletes must be deliberate and conscientious in their athletic progression. Pushing things too fast, as the hare learned the hard way, can yield below par and unexpected results. Youngsters should first become gradually initiated to exercise, proceed by building a foundation of strength, conditioning, and athleticism, and finally move on to full-scale performance enhancement training and sport specialization.

Specializing too early (Phases 1 and 2) can cause a myriad of problems, such as overuse injuries, burnout, and the loss of biological equilibrium. And there is no proof that early specialization is a precursor to future sports success. In fact, many studies seem to suggest just the opposite: that a long-term, balanced approach to participation and training leads to more athletic prosperity later in one's development. To illustrate this point, study the career of NFL legend Jim Brown. In high school, this phenomenal athlete was not only an All-American football running back, but averaged 38 points on the basketball team his senior year, ran track, played baseball, and is still to this day considered to be perhaps the greatest lacrosse player ever to pick up a stick—quite the poster athlete for balanced sports training.

4. Supervision

With the exception of training sessions that include only late Phase 3 athletes, all youth strength and conditioning workouts should be supervised by an experienced adult. The reasons for this are numerous with the first and foremost being safety. Having a supervisor on hand will ensure that proper exercise/drill execution is adhered to at all times, make certain fatigue levels of participants are monitored regularly, discourage any type of horseplay from taking place, and generally engender a safe training environment. Attention to safety, while important for all age groups, is especially necessary when supervising Phase 1 children who, as mentioned earlier in the chapter, have a tendency to lose concentration during workouts.

A competent, knowledgeable supervisor provides another important function. He contributes toward increasing workout productivity, allowing youngsters to garner the most out of their training sessions. Some of the ways a supervisor will accomplish this function include maintaining workout continuity and pace, providing encouragement and motivation, and being available to answer relevant workout-related questions. Some dedicated supervisors will even take time to personally analyze a youngster's progress and make suggestions for improvement.

5. Beware of Burnout

Burnout (unfortunately) has become synonymous with youth sports over the past decade or so. Despite the overall number of participants in youth sports rising substantially throughout the United States, most estimates claim that in the neighborhood of 70 percent of youngsters will quit playing organized sports by age 13. Not all, of course, will be suffering from burnout. Many youngsters simply decide to move on to other interests. However, a troubling sign is that even many promising early teen athletes are expressing that sports is becoming more of a burden than a joy.

Theories abound as to why burnout rates are so high. One points to the feverish season after season schedule to which many young athletes adhere. Between regular seasons, off-season tournaments, and showcase-oriented summer camps, children as young seven or eight already have full plates of year-round sports activities.

Another is the trend toward early specialization. An alarming number of young athletes are erroneously pushed into one sport at the expense of all others. This lack of variety causes many youngsters to lose interest. Early specialization also leaves young athletes vulnerable to injury, because performing the same movements week after week, month after month, and year after year takes its toll on their still developing bodies. Chronic injuries are extremely frustrating, and ultimately force many youngsters to the sideline indefinitely.

Performance pressure is also cited as cause for burnout. Making this situation worse is that the greatest pressure most often comes from parents. The failure to live up to performance expectations—especially from the people closest to the youngster—can lead to feelings of inadequacy and futility, which are not exactly the feelings that will keep youngsters involved in sporting activities.

Incorporating the information in *Peak Conditioning Training for Young Athletes* can help youngsters avoid burning out. Paying more attention to general, year-round fitness (as opposed to relentless sports competition) may be at least one way to lower the incidence of burnout among young athletes. A reasonable balance between skill development, competition, and fitness training is just what the doctor ordered (and many of them do) when it comes to preventing burnout.

6. Overtraining

Overtraining is the enemy of all athletes, and young athletes are no exception. It hinders performance, stymies improvement, and often leads to injury. Because of their less-developed and ever-growing bodies—not to mention their hectic sports and life schedules—young athletes are often more susceptible to this debilitating condition than are their older, physically mature counterparts. As such, achieving the delicate balance between training and rest for youngsters is an extremely challenging proposition, one that must be addressed seriously and regularly if athletic potential is to be reached.

Thankfully, good news is on the horizon concerning overtraining for young athletes. Advances in exercise physiology and the increased availability of competent trainers and youth coaches has lowered the incidence of overtraining considerably among young athletes in recent years. Therefore, with careful planning and mindful attention (and by following the suggestions and training programs in *Peak Conditioning Training for Young Athletes*) youngsters can, for the most part, avoid this frustrating state. Of course, youth coaches, program directors, fitness trainers, and parents must be constantly on the alert for signs of overtraining in the youngsters under their auspices. Most young athletes, especially Phase 1 children, have not yet developed an intuitive feel for how their bodies are responding to exercise, so it is up to adults to remain hyper-vigilant in this area. For their part, young athletes should make clear to the coaches, parents, and fitness trainers how they are feeling from a physical standpoint on a regular basis.

Major Symptoms of Overtraining

- Noticeable loss of strength, power, and conditioning
- Increased muscle, joint, and tendon soreness
- Lack of enthusiasm for workouts
- A preponderance of minor injuries
- Insomnia
- Decrease in appetite
- General irritability (Teenagers, of course, don't need to be overtrained to be irritable!)

Proven Remedies for Young Athletes Who Suffer from Overtraining

- Take a break from training (one to two weeks).
- Decrease the intensity of workouts.
- Change up exercise routine.
- Include some extra stretching and warm-up/cool-down activities.
- Make sure that a balanced, calorie-sufficient diet is consumed on a daily basis.

If the symptoms of overtraining persist for two weeks or more, be sure to see a sports medicine physician.

7. Differences Between Boys and Girls

Most experienced youth coaches, trainers, and program directors are well aware of the differences between girls and boys as they mature and grow. The overwhelming majority of girls mature physically much earlier than do boys. Growth spurts in girls can take place as early as age 10 or 11 and top off at age 12 or 13, just prior to the beginning of menstruation. Boys, on the other hand, hit their main growth spurt anywhere from 13 to 15 years of age. In most cases, boys catch up to and eventually surpass girls in terms of physical development.

Adults who work regularly with female athletes in the 10 to 13 age range should note that some in the medical community discourage intense physical activity during this period. They suggest that girls who commence hard physical training in the prepubescent years may delay the onset of menarche (first occurrence of menstruation in women). Late onset can compromise bone health and other growth related functions. Research in this area has not been definitive, however, and other factors other than exercise, such as diet and individual genetics must be also be taken into account. Nevertheless, all female athletes in this age group should regularly schedule visits with their physicians to discuss and monitor the effects of a heavy sports training schedule.

8. Limit Performance Pressure

Young athletes are under tremendous pressure to succeed in this day and age. The win-at-all-cost mentality has ratcheted its way down to youth sports, making once simple and enjoyable activities into do-or-die events for many.

It must be clearly understood by all youth coaches, program directors, and parents that young athletes are not only developing physically, but emotionally as well. They are not emotionally ready to handle high degrees of outside performance pressure, any more than they would be physically ready to handle Michael Jordan's workout routine. Applying too much pressure to a youngster to succeed in sports (or anything else for that matter) will usually have the opposite effect and actually hinder performance. Moreover, long-term problems such as perfectionism or competition avoidance can often be traced to youngsters who were pushed too hard to win and succeed on the playing field.

9. Physical Training is a Year-Round Proposition

Similar to their older counterparts, young athletes should approach physical training from a year-round perspective. Training periodically, say six weeks prior to an upcoming season, is certainly better than not preparing at all. However, for best results, an exercise regime should be adhered to on a year-round basis. Conditioning the body throughout the year assures that a reasonable level of fitness will be maintained at all times. This practice will allow the youngster to peak for seasons and competitions in a gradual and efficient manner without overtraining which often occurs when the conditioning process is rushed.

10. Everybody is an Athlete

While this book is geared toward those youngsters who aspire to improve performance in sports, you need not be an "athlete" to benefit from working out. Studies have shown that early teens who exercise regularly tend to have higher levels of self esteem, and are less likely to smoke, drink, take drugs, be overweight, or drop out of school. Additionally, the health and exercise habits developed at young ages usually continue throughout life, helping athletes and non-athletes alike live longer, healthier, and more productive lives.

2

Warm-Up, Cool-Down, and Flexibility

Warming up, cooling down, and stretching regularly are key components of a balanced youth sports conditioning program. They are also essential prerequisites for all young athletes seeking to reach their full athletic potential.

Warm-Up

Warming up prior to any type of intense physical activity—be it a sports competition, team practice, or conditioning workout—is a three-fold process. It will include some type of light exertion such as riding a stationary bicycle or running in place for five to eight minutes, followed by a comprehensive stretching routine like the one detailed later in this chapter, and culminating with low-intensity involvement in the desired activity (i.e., high repetition sets of weightlifting or striding at a medium pace prior to sprinting). Warming up correctly contributes to productive workouts, enhanced sports performance, and (most importantly) the prevention of injuries. All young athletes, regardless of phase or sport, should make the warm-up a regular part of their sports improvement program.

Cool-Down

The cool-down process consists of a few minutes of low-intensity activity similar to the first step of the warm-up, followed by an abbreviated flexibility session that focuses on stretching the lower back, hamstrings, and shoulders. Actively cooling down after high-intensity exertion will help the body recover for the next competition/workout, along with allowing it to return to its naturally relaxed state faster, thus promoting physiological balance and sound sleep. An example of the warm-up/cool-down continuum is detailed in Table 2-1.

Warm-Up Phase 1–Low-Intensity Activity
Perform five to eight minutes of light exercise, such as running in place, stationary biking, or slow-paced jogging. This type of activity raises your body temperature and gets the blood flowing to your muscles, which will allow you to stretch (phase 2) through a greater range of motion.

Prepares the body for

Warm-Up Phase 2–Flexibility Training
12 to 20 stretches (detailed in the next section)

Prepares the body for

Warm-Up Phase 3–Medium-Intensity Involvement in Desired Activity
Examples: Strength training—two light, high repetition (15 to 20) sets
Plyometric training—low-intensity bounding
Agility training—jumping rope at medium speed

Prepares the body for

Intense All-Out Activity

Cool-Down Phase 1–Low-Intensity Activity (See Warm-Up Phase 1)
Cool-Down Phase 2–Abbreviated Flexibility Routine
Six to eight stretches with an emphasis on the lower back, hamstrings, and shoulders.

Table 2-1. Warm-up/cool-down continuum

Flexibility Training

It's no secret that, to the majority of young athletes, stretching is nothing more than a necessary nuisance, something they are forced to do by conscientious coaches and trainers. Most reason that because their young bodies are so inherently limber, especially when compared to older, physically mature athletes, they would be much better served using the 12 to 15 minutes of stretching time in the weight room pumping iron, or, better yet, out on the field or court practicing their favorite sport.

This line of thinking is, of course, erroneous. All serious athletes, regardless of age, level, or physical maturity should engage in a comprehensive, year-round flexibility program, one that includes a variety of stretches and is performed both before and after all intense physical activities. The most important athletic benefits of consistent flexibility training include that it:

- Readies the body for intense physical activity
- Promotes optimal athletic performance and productive workouts
- Enhances recovery from workouts and competitions
- Helps to prevent injury
- Increases strength, speed, explosiveness, and quickness
- Prolongs athletic careers
- Engenders discipline

Before moving on to the different types of stretching techniques and the flexibility routines themselves, it is important to at least briefly address the challenging proposition of convincing young athletes to stretch. The one (and in my experience, only) strategy for successfully encouraging youngsters to stretch regularly is for coaches, trainers, parents, and anyone else involved in a young athlete's conditioning activities to strongly emphasize the performance-enhancing by-products of flexibility training such as increasing speed, improving strength, and enhancing jumping ability. The fact is that most youngsters are not overly interested in faster recovery from workouts, prolonging their athletic careers, or even preventing injuries (until they have one, that is). But if they recognize a direct correlation between stretching consistently and hitting more home runs, scoring more touchdowns, or sinking more baskets, they are more likely to get down on the stretching mat on a daily basis. A variety of different stretching methods are available to youngsters. The five following are the most popular.

Static Stretching

Static stretching will be the mainstay of a young athletes flexibility routine. It entails slowly stretching a muscle to the point of slight discomfort (not pain) and holding the stretch for 20 to 50 seconds. Static stretching, along with being extremely effective, is the safest of all stretching techniques. The flexibility program to follow consists of a variety of static stretches.

Ballistic Stretching

Ballistic stretching has experienced a resurgence in recent years throughout the sports strength and conditioning community. (It was regularly used decades ago before it fell out of favor.) Ballistic stretching incorporates a series of dynamic, bouncing movements when stretching a muscle group. While the method has shown to increase flexibility in some, many feel that the abrupt muscle contractions may put developing young athletes at risk of injury. Therefore, youngsters should use ballistic stretching with caution. If a young athlete chooses to experiment with this stretching technique, he must first make sure that all muscles are sufficiently warmed up prior to beginning. In fact, many conditioning experts suggest that a full static stretching routine be completed before any ballistic movements are executed. For obvious reasons, injured athletes should not use ballistic stretching.

Passive Partner-Assisted Stretching

Passive partner-assisted stretching calls for a partner to add light pressure to each static stretch. This technique has shown to increase joint and muscle range of motion when performed regularly. For best (and safe) results, the assisting partner should be an adult with experience in teaching flexibility methods.

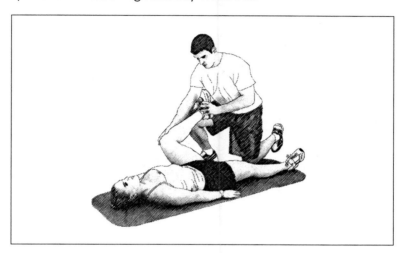

Proprioceptive Neuromuscular Facilitation (PNF) Stretching

Proprioceptive neuromuscular facilitation (PNF) stretching is not quite as complicated as the name sounds. It involves a partner/facilitator leading a young athlete through a series of positions (contract, hold, relax, and movement) in 10-second intervals. If executed correctly, this technique (used by numerous professional athletes in a variety of sports) can substantially increase joint and muscle flexibility. Unfortunately, the majority of junior high schools and high schools—not to mention grammar schools—do not have individuals on staff who are experienced with PNF techniques. Incorrect execution of this method can cause serious injury. As such, PNF stretching should only be incorporated in a youth flexibility program if the appropriate assisting personnel are available on a regular basis.

Rope-/Strap-Assisted Stretching

Rope-/strap-assisted stretching is similar to PNF and passive partner assisted stretching in that it allows young athletes to take their muscles and joints through a greater range of motion. Unlike the two previously detailed techniques, however, a partner/facilitator is not required, so youngsters can stretch on their own. This method entails grasping one end of the rope or strap with both hands and attaching the other end to the appropriate area of the body (foot, ankle, elbow, etc.). From there, the young athlete will pull on the rope/strap with the appropriate force in order to stretch the muscle.

Although a stretching rope/strap is relatively simple to use, a learning curve does exist. Therefore, all youngsters should seek out an experienced practitioner to help them master correct form before incorporating this equipment into their flexibility training. If a strap or rope is not available, a rolled up towel can be substituted.

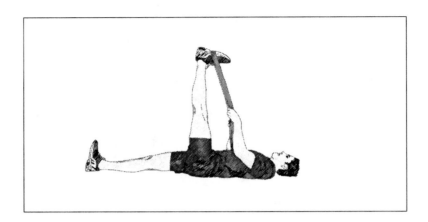

Flexibility Program

The following flexibility program details a stretching workout that is appropriate for young athletes in all phases of development. The entire routine can be accomplished in 15 to 20 minutes, and should be performed on a year-round basis, both before and after strenuous athletic activity. With slight variations, many of the following stretches can be performed ballistically, partner assisted, or with a stretching rope or strap. As young athletes progress and become more flexible and experienced, they are encouraged to add and subtract individual stretches as they see fit.

1. *Knees to Chest*
- Lie flat on your back with your legs extended.
- Grasp your upper shins just below your kneecaps and pull your knees to your chest. Hold for 30 seconds.
- Alternate by pulling one leg at a time while keeping the other leg extended on the floor. Hold for 20 seconds.
- Perform four sets—two sets with both legs and one set each with alternating legs.

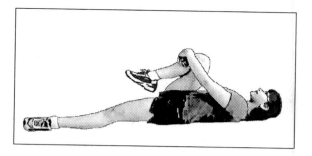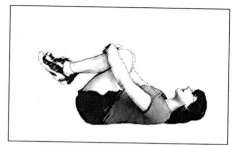

2. Back Arch

- Lie flat on your back with your legs extended.
- Flex your knees, sliding your feet toward your buttocks, and lift your pelvis off the floor while arching your back.
- Perform one set holding in an arched position for 50 seconds.

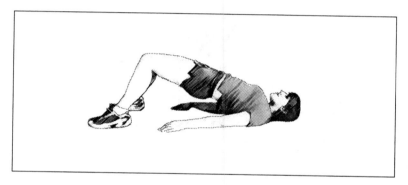

3. Hip Flexor Stretch

- Lie flat on your back with your knees flexed and your hands clasped behind your neck.
- Slowly lower both knees to the floor, keeping your head, shoulders, and elbows flat on the floor. Hold at the bottom position for 20 seconds.
- Perform two sets for each side.

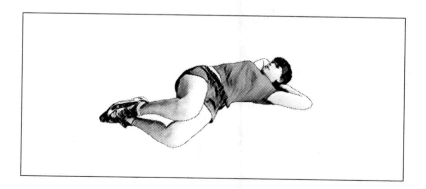

4. *Lying Hamstring Stretch*

- Lie flat on your back with your legs flexed and your heels close to your buttocks.
- Extend one leg upward and grasp underneath it. Then, slowly pull it toward you while keeping the other leg planted on the floor. Hold for 20 seconds.
- Perform two sets with each leg.

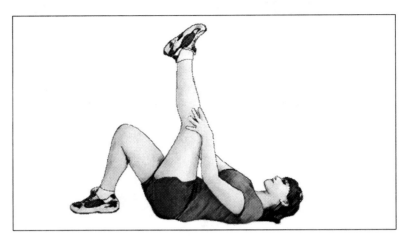

5. *Standing Hamstring Stretch*

- Stand erect with your feet close together.
- Maintaining straight legs, bend forward at the waist, and touch your toes.
- Hold for 30 seconds.
- Perform two sets.

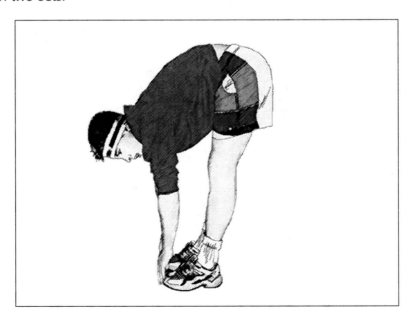

6. *Reverse Plough*

- Lie face down on the floor with your body extended.
- Place your palms on the floor between your chest and your hips.
- Press down evenly, and raise your head and trunk straight upward. Hold for 30 seconds.
- Perform two sets.

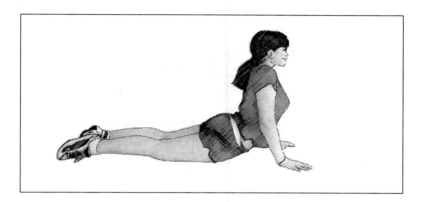

7. *Plough to Seated Hamstring Stretch*

- Lie flat on your back with your arms on your hips.
- Raise both slightly bent legs up over your head and slowly lower your feet to the floor.
- After holding the stretch for 30 seconds, return under control to the seated position with your legs extended directly in front of you.
- Keeping both legs straight, bend forward at the waist and slowly lower your trunk to your thighs, while simultaneously reaching your hands to your toes. Hold for 30 seconds.
- Perform two sets.

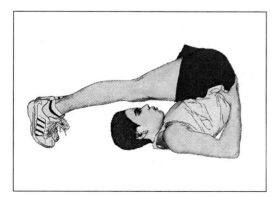
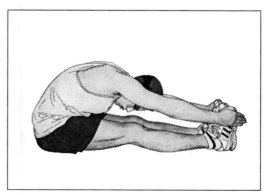

8. *Lower Back/Quadriceps Stretch*

- Lie face down on the floor with your body extended.
- Reach back and grab both ankles.
- Pull your ankles toward your upper back while at the same time lifting your chest off the floor. Hold for 45 seconds.
- Perform one set.

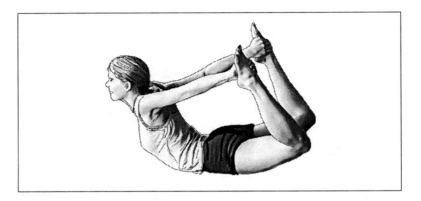

9. *Bar Hang*

- With a shoulder width, overhand grip and arms extended hang from a chinning bar. Hang for 30 seconds.
- Perform two sets.

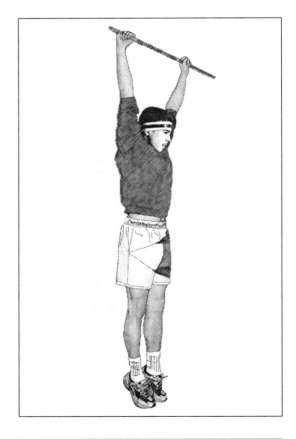

10. *Kneeling Low Back Stretch*

- Kneel on all fours on the floor.
- Contract your abdominal muscles while simultaneously rounding your back. Hold for 30 seconds.
- Perform two sets.

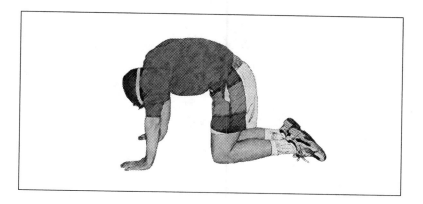

11. *Seated Groin Stretch*

- Sit upright on the floor.
- Bend your knees and bring your feet together and then pull them toward you from the lower shins. Hold for 20 seconds.
- Perform two sets.

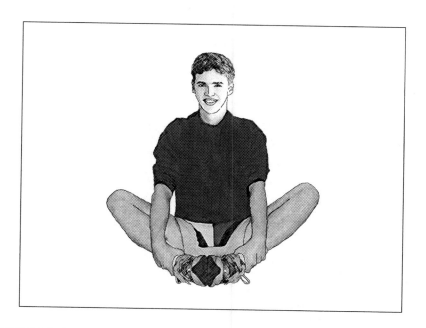

12. *Standing Groin Stretch*

- Stand with your legs spread approximately twice as wide as your shoulders.
- Bend straight down and attempt to touch your fingertips to the floor. Hold for 30 seconds.
- Perform two sets.

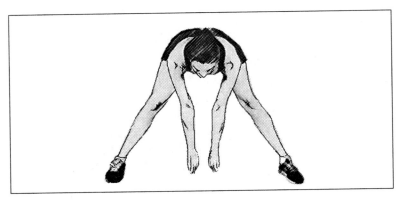

13. *Standing Quadriceps Stretch*

- Stand upright, bracing yourself with one hand against a wall for balance.
- Reach down and grasp one foot (right hand/right foot; left hand/left foot).
- Pull your heel to your buttocks and hold for 20 seconds.
- Perform two sets with each leg.

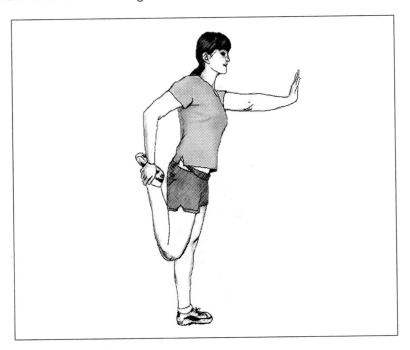

14. *Calf Stretch*

- Stand upright with both hands against a wall and your arms fully extended.
- Lean forward with your feet remaining flat on the floor, bending your arms and stretching your calves. Hold for 30 seconds.
- Perform two sets.

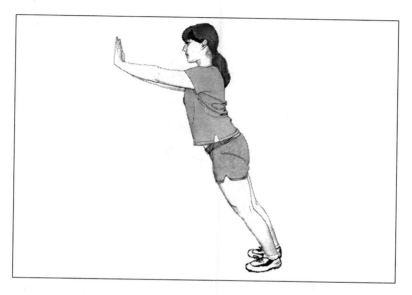

15. *Hands Clasped Shoulder Stretch*

- Stand upright and cross one wrist over the other and interlock your hands.
- With your arms extended behind your head, shrug your shoulders upwards and reach toward the ceiling. Hold for 30 seconds.
- Perform two sets with hands clasped each way.

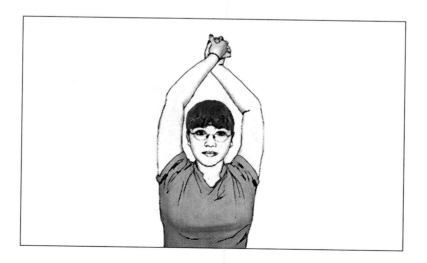

16. *Lateral Shoulder Stretch*

- Sit upright on a flat back chair or exercise bench.
- Pull your arm at the elbow across your opposite shoulder. Hold for 30 seconds.
- Perform two sets for each arm.

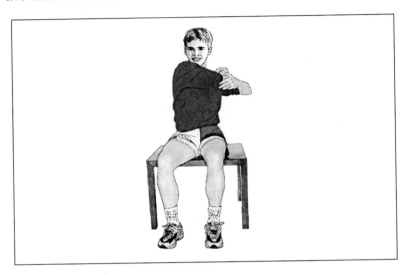

17. *Upper Back Stretch*

- Stand erect with your feet approximately six inches apart at arms length from a bar or other supporting object.
- Maintaining straight arms and legs, bend at the waist, flatten your back, and grab hold of the bar/supporting object with both hands.
- Press down by extending your shoulders and arching your back. Hold for 30 seconds.
- Perform two sets.

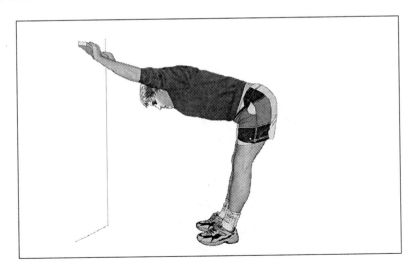

18. *Chest Stretch*

- Stand erect facing an open doorway.
- Bend both arms at the elbow and raise them approximately six inches above head height.
- Lean your entire body forward, bracing your weight on the outside of the doorway, and stretch your chest. Hold for 30 seconds.
- Perform two sets.

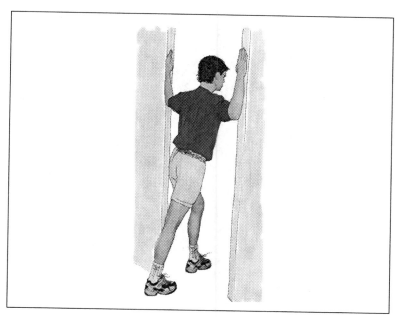

19. *Triceps Stretch*

- Sit or stand with one arm flexed and raised overhead next to your ear. Rest your hand on your shoulder blade.
- Grasp your elbow with the opposite hand and pull it behind your head. Hold for 20 seconds.
- Perform two sets with each arm.

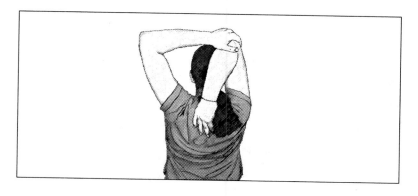

20. *Neck Rolls*

- Roll your neck in deliberate fashion first clockwise then counter clockwise. Continue for 20 seconds.
- Perform one set in each direction.

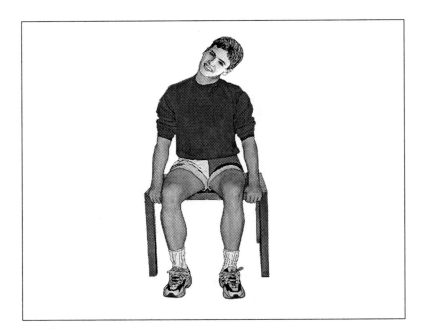

Pre-Movement Training Exercises

Prior to all movement-oriented workouts (speed, agility, plyometrics, etc.), it is imperative that, along with the conventional warm-up and stretching activities discussed earlier, youngsters perform the following series of pre-movement training exercises. These medium-intensity drills will set the stage for the high-intensity movement training to follow.

Exercise: Leg Swings

Execution: Stand sideways to a wall or bar and brace yourself against it with your inside hand. With your outside hand relaxed at your side and your outside leg planted firmly on the ground, swing your inside leg straight in front of your body and then back behind your body.

Sets and Repetitions: Two sets of 20 repetitions with each leg

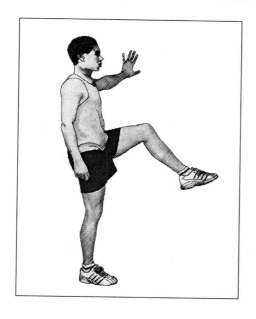
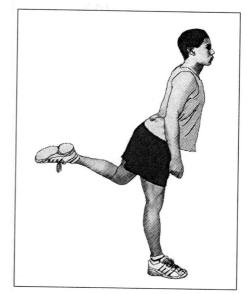

Exercise: Side Kicks

Execution: Stand facing a wall or bar and brace both of your slightly bent arms against it. With your knee flexed slightly, proceed to swing your left leg from side to side, while keeping your right leg planted firmly on the floor. Repeat with your right leg.

Sets and Repetitions: Two sets of 15 repetitions with each leg

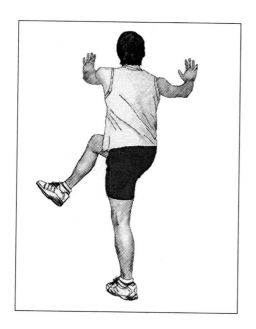
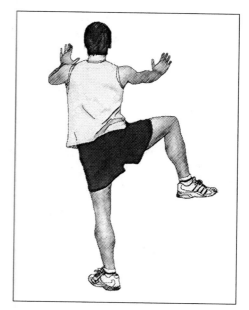

Exercise: Butt Kicks

Execution: Run straight ahead at an easy pace, attempting to kick your heels toward your buttocks.

Sets and Repetitions: Two sets of 20 yards

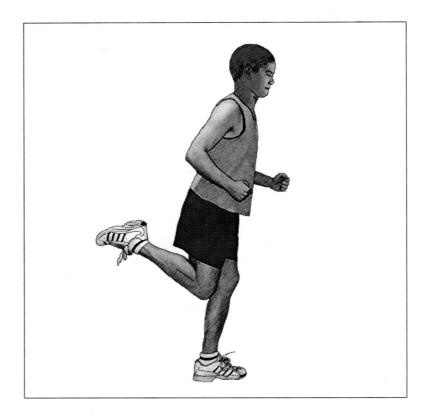

Exercise: Body-Weight Side Lunge

Executions: Standing straight with your hands relaxed at your sides, step laterally, bend at the knees, and bring your back knee close to the floor. Proceed to drive yourself back up to the standing position.

Sets and Repetitions: Two sets of 20 repetitions with each leg

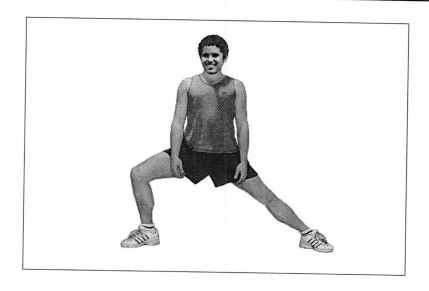

Exercise: Backpedals

Execution: With a slight forward lean and your back straight, backpedal on the balls of your feet using short, choppy strides. Your head should be up, eyes fixed straight ahead, and arms positioned close to your body and at approximately chest height.

Sets and Repetitions: Four sets of 15 yards

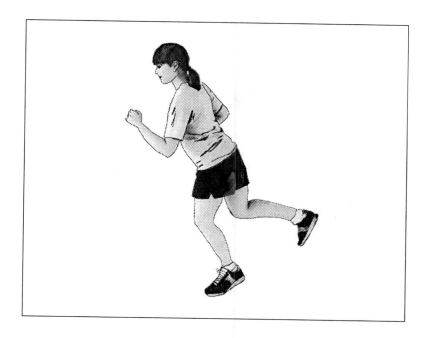

Exercise: Carioca

Execution: Begin in an athletic stance—head up, back straight, legs slightly wider than shoulder width, and knees flexed. Proceed to step laterally with your left foot. Follow immediately by stepping behind your left foot with your right foot, while simultaneously turning your hips in the direction you want to go. From there, push your right leg powerfully in front of your left leg and continue in this pattern for the required distance. Change direction and repeat.

Sets and Repetitions: Four sets of 20 yards in each direction

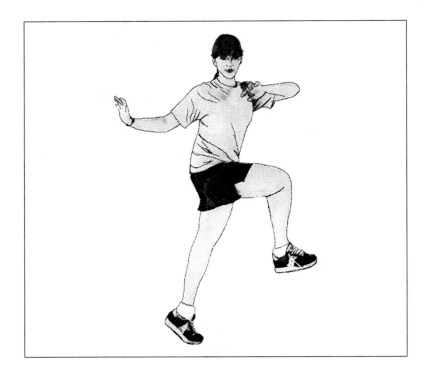

Exercise: Tin Soldier

Execution: From a standing position, proceed to kick your left leg straight up (no knee flex) while simultaneously extending your left arm directly forward. Your toes should lightly graze your fingertips at the top. When your left leg returns to the ground, execute the same movement with your right leg and right arm as you step forward. Continue in this pattern for the required distance.

Sets and Repetitions: Four sets of 12 yards each

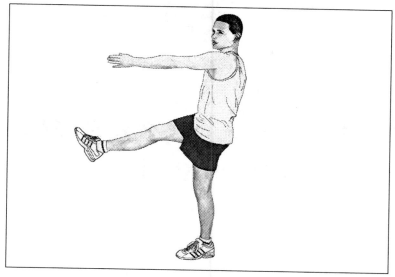

Exercise: Three-Quarter-Speed Bound

Execution: Begin by striding forward at a deliberate pace for 10 yards. At the 10-yard mark, proceed to jump off your left foot at 75 percent of maximum, while simultaneously lifting your right knee as if executing a basketball lay-up. Your arms will rise up in unison to just above head height. Let your momentum carry you forward. Land under control on the jumping leg (the left leg in this example), and repeat the process, but this time jump and land with the right leg. The concentration on all bounding drills should be on jumping up rather than out.

Sets and Repetitions: Two sets of 30 yards (not including the initial 10 yards of striding)

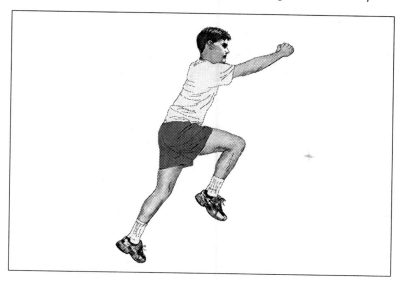

3

Recuperation, Sleep, Attitude, and Injuries

If young athletes are to perform at peak levels on a year-round basis, they must take adequate time to recover between exercises, workouts, and training cycles; garner sufficient amounts of sound sleep; maintain a positive attitude; and deal conscientiously with injuries. The following are ways to achieve these worthwhile objectives.

Recuperation

Giving the body the opportunity to adequately recover from the rigors of training and competition is a prerequisite for sports success. Unfortunately, recuperation is a very tricky subject, since no two young athletes have exactly the same recovery needs. Some are able to bounce back remarkably quickly from even the most strenuous physical workouts, while others respond best by employing maximum rest intervals between bouts of exercise. Still others, the majority, fall somewhere in-between. Needless to say, proper recuperation necessitates a very individual and delicate balance.

While coaches, trainers, experienced teammates, and well-meaning parents can steer young athletes in the right direction when it comes to their recovery requirements, it is ultimately up to the youngster himself to develop an intuitive feel for when to push ahead with hard training and when to ease off. This approach may seem like a lot to ask of a young, inexperienced athlete, but taking personal responsibility is the first and most important step toward divining individual recovery needs. All elite athletes can tell from day to day (if not hour to hour) whether their bodies are best served by more or less work. The earlier youngsters can learn to do this, the more successful their athletic careers will ultimately be.

Sleep

A counselor at a popular youth sports camp once said, "If you want to soar with the eagles in the daytime, you can't hoot with the owls at night." Sound words. A hard-training young athlete must get adequate sleep and rest if he hopes to perform at his best. Sleep requirements vary, sometimes considerably, from youngster to youngster. Some are able to get by on very little with no ill effects. Others need substantial rack time in order to maintain peak performance levels.

On average, Phase 1 children will need ten to ten-and-a-half hours of sleep per night, Phase 2 youngsters nine to ten hours, and Phase 3 athletes seven-and-a-half to nine hours. Short naps (20 to 30 minutes) in the middle of the day can help to rejuvenate young athletes and should be incorporated for those who have the time and inclination. Longer naps (two to three hours) tend to cause grogginess and therefore should be avoided, especially on competition days.

Sleep researchers suggest that waking up at the same time every day regardless of when the prior night's bedtime was is helpful in developing a regular sleep pattern. This habit may be difficult at times for young athletes, especially after late night competitions or workouts, but it is a proven strategy for improving the quality of sleep and should be adhered to whenever possible.

Coffee and other highly caffeinated products such as colas and chocolate should be kept to a minimum, especially late in the day, as these substances can cause insomnia. Excess sugar intake also contributes to keeping youngsters up at night, thus sugary snacks should be avoided after lunchtime (and altogether if possible).

On the other hand, warm milk and soft cheeses consumed close to bedtime can improve sleep quality. Other popular sleep remedies include stretching deliberately in the early evening and taking a warm bath or whirlpool two to three hours before turning in.

Two notoriously difficult times for young athletes to garner a good night's sleep are the night before an important competition and the night after participating in a late day or night sporting event. The key to sleeping well the night before a competition, say a playoff game, is more mental than it is physical. This doesn't mean, of course, that youngsters shouldn't follow suggestions such as taking a warm bath, drinking some warm milk, and avoiding caffeine close to bedtime. However, getting the mind off of tomorrow's responsibilities is the real secret to entering pre-competition dreamland.

After practice/training is concluded on the day before competition, it's time to stop thinking about the following day's sports activities. Young athletes are encouraged to go to a movie, read a non-sports related book, watch some mindless television (not too hard for kids these days), or anything to keep their minds off of the upcoming competition. Thinking incessantly about what's going to happen on the field, court, or track the next day will do absolutely nothing to improve athletic performance. In fact, the sleep sacrificed by obsessing about tomorrow's athletic duties will actually hinder the ability to execute.

Now, on to the even more challenging proposition of sleeping after a late day or night competition. Here youngsters will not only encounter the psychological aspect of dwelling on their performance, which many elite athletes describe as a movie repeating itself frame-by-frame over and over and over again, but the physiological ramifications as well.

Coping with the mental side of the equation of sleeping after competitions basically mirrors that of the pre-competition nights, with the only difference being that instead of endeavoring to keep the mind off what is going to be done, young athletes will be attempting to block out repetitively re-living what they've just accomplished (on the playing field, court, ice, track, etc.). Use the same methods previously described to refrain from dwelling on past competition performance, whether it was good, bad, or mediocre. Easier said than done, of course, but these techniques are necessary to attain that elusive post-competition shut-eye.

Let's now switch our attention to the physiological aspect of sleeping after late day or night competitions. The body will likely be in overdrive after an intense competition. Competitive action elicits a high level of adrenaline flow, which unfortunately doesn't leave the body when the event concludes. It can literally take hours for the system to work its way back to a normal, balanced state. However, some strategies can be implemented that will contribute to cycling down the young body after a hard fought competition. Three of the most helpful strategies are presented as follows.

Engage in a Comprehensive Post-Game Cool-Down

As discussed in Chapter 2, cooling down efficiently after intense physical exertion is extremely important. Subsequent to a late day or night competition, it is absolutely critical, especially when it comes to getting a good night's rest. Following the cool-down protocol discussed in Chapter 2 should help considerably in the quest for sound post-competition slumber.

Hit the Weight Room After Competition

Heading to the weight room immediately following participating in a sporting event is not only a great way to maintain in-season strength and power, but it also contributes to pumping some of that competition induced adrenaline out of the system. Many professional sports teams require that their athletes lift after all games. Youngsters should be encouraged to do the same if the appropriate facilities are available. Post-competition strength workouts should be relatively brief (30 to 35 minutes at most), and must include high levels of fluid consumption before, during, and after the training sessions.

Eat a Healthy, Filling Post-Competition Meal

After a competition, it will have been a number of hours since a young athlete has last eaten. (Most pre-competition meals take place three to four hours before an event.) Going to bed on an empty stomach after competition is a sure ticket to disrupted sleep—not to mention depleted energy stores for the following day's activities. As such, a substantial post-competition meal should be eaten within two-and-a-half to three hours after the conclusion of a late event. For more detailed information about post-competition eating, refer to Chapter 4.

Maintain a Positive Attitude

Like life, sports has its fair share of ups and downs. Wins and productive competitions are interspersed with losses and below par performances. No matter how talented a young athlete is or how hard he works, failure will periodically follow him on to the field, court, or track. It's inevitable.

The same holds true in a strength and conditioning program. Not all workouts are created equal. Some will be satisfying and improvement promoting. Others will be lackluster and disappointing. Sticking points in training, minor injuries, and unexpected changes in schedule are all frustrating realities for athletes young and old alike.

The ability to bounce back from bad competitions and workouts is a key factor to success in sports. Learning how to transcend circumstances and maintain a positive, improvement-conscious attitude when the chips are down is of paramount importance for all young athletes. Following are some tips for keeping up a positive attitude when things aren't going as planned.

Be Aware

Remaining mindful of disappointments and frustrations is essential for all young athletes. They may have left the tying run on base, missed an important free throw, or lost a running race they were expecting to win. The specific transgression matters not. Awareness is the first step in dealing with adversity. Once it is taken, moving on is possible.

Analyze Briefly

Youngsters should analyze their sports failures briefly (emphasis on briefly), learn what they can from them, and move on. Dwelling on mistakes is a waste of time and energy. Approaching sports related up and downs in this manner will help young athletes become clear-minded and ultimately better performers.

Focus on the Future

Focusing intensely on the next task after experiencing a sports disappointment is crucial to maintaining a positive, winning attitude. Most top athletes from a variety of sports find that "setting their minds forward" allows them to move past inevitable failures quickly and proceed to perform at their best.

Remember, Nobody's Perfect

Most dedicated young athletes demand a lot of themselves. They work hard and strive for perfection. However, striving for perfection is one thing; actually achieving perfection is quite another. Perfection (unfortunately) is not a human trait. Even the most exemplary athletes experience failure and make mistakes regularly. Youth coaches, trainers, and especially parents should be very clear in letting young athletes know that perfection in any given sport is not expected or possible.

Injuries

As the popularity, competition, and time spent participating has increased in youth sports so, not surprisingly, has the number of injuries. Overuse injuries such as tendonitis and stress fractures are the major culprits with over eight million young athletes experiencing them each year. Dynamic impact related injuries (ligament tears, broken bones, separated shoulders, etc.) are also on the rise, as competitions, team practices, and off-season workouts become ever more demanding and physical.

Injury Prevention

The key to avoiding injury for young athletes lies first and foremost with proper prevention. "An ounce of prevention is worth a pound of cure," as the old saying goes, and truer words were never spoken when it comes to sports-related injuries. Fortunately, with the advances in strength, conditioning, and nutrition in recent years, many sports injuries can be averted or, at the very least, significantly curtailed. The following are a variety of strategies young athletes can implement to help stave off injury.

Strength train regularly. Of all aspects of physical conditioning, strength training is far and away the most important when it comes to the prevention of injury. The additional strength youngsters build around their joints and throughout their bodies reduces stress considerably during repetitive actions such as pitching a baseball or softball, swinging a tennis racket, or jogging long distances. Stronger, more powerful youngsters also are able to absorb the shock of high-impact contact and forceful twisting motions that occur frequently in sports such as football, hockey, and lacrosse. Finally, a strong, well-developed core (mid-section, lower back, hips) will help youngsters stave off numerous lower back ailments, which as any athlete who has experienced debilitating lower back pain can attest, usually results in extended downtime from sporting and workout-related activities. Chapters 6, 7, and 8 cover all phases of youth strength training in detail.

Stretch, stretch, stretch. Stretching both before and after any type of intense physical activity will be emphasized again and again throughout this book. Why? It's simply that important, especially when it comes to preventing a myriad of injuries. Readers should refer regularly to Chapter 2 for complete and comprehensive coverage of flexibility training.

Sleep. Sleep mentally and physically rejuvenates the young athlete. Those who do not get enough of it not only perform below their capabilities, but put themselves at a much higher risk for injury. Many, if not most, sports and workout-related injuries occur when an athlete's body is in a weakened state. Lack of sound sleep on a regular basis contributes mightily to a weakened bodily state.

Eat well. As with getting sufficient sleep, adhering to a balanced, nutritionally sound diet helps the young body stay strong, conditioned, and healthy. Possessing these attributes goes a long way toward preventing injury. See Chapter 4 for detailed information about youth sports nutrition.

Avoid overtraining. Overtraining (and its effects on the young athlete) was discussed in Chapter 1. Youngsters who are overtrained are perpetually tired. Most injuries, whether they occur on the playing field, in the weight room, or during a conditioning workout are a byproduct of the athlete being physically fatigued and worn down.

Injury Rehabilitation

Despite the high level of physical conditioning most serious young athletes attain today, injuries are still an inevitable part of sports. In fact, it is virtually impossible for even the most highly conditioned young athlete to escape injury forever. The following are a variety of rehabilitation tips that youngsters can employ to make their journey from injury to activity a little easier. Keep in mind that the following information is not meant in any way to take the place of consulting and working closely with experienced medical and rehabilitation personnel.

Let them know. When a youngster sustains an injury of any kind during sports or workout activities, the first step is to immediately communicate with the appropriate individuals (coaches, trainers, parents, doctors, etc.). A clear and succinct explanation of an injury is crucial to proper diagnosis and a key to quick recovery. Doctors and trainers, while experienced in dealing with injured athletes, are far from mind readers. As such, parents and coaches should encourage young athletes to be as precise as possible when describing an injury. Doing so will go a long way toward ensuring that the suitable treatment/rehabilitation protocol will be prescribed.

Choose the right physical therapist. Once an injured young athlete is examined by a doctor, it is time to go about the process of choosing a physical therapist to help with the rehabilitation. While all professional sports franchises and most college programs have highly-trained rehabilitation personnel on staff, the large majority of high schools and junior high schools—not to mention grammar schools—do not. Therefore it will more than likely be up to parents to do the footwork themselves when it comes to finding an appropriate therapist for their injured son or daughter.

Just like doctors, physical therapists tend to specialize in specific injuries. As such, the first step in narrowing down the choices is to locate those therapists in the area who deal regularly and competently with the injury in question.

From there, it's time to seek recommendations. A few of the best sources for physical therapist recommendations include athletes who've sustained similar injuries, coaches and athletic trainers in the area, and school nurses.

Next comes the facility visit, which will allow the young athlete and his parents to get a feel for the workout space. Is it well equipped? Spacious? Cramped? Pay particular attention to the atmosphere within the training area, since rehabilitation workouts will take all the enthusiasm a youngster can muster. Also, make sure that the therapist you choose is not spread too thin among patients. One-on-one attention is crucial to a successful patient therapist relationship, especially in the beginning stages of rehabilitation.

Finally, once a choice has been made, try to stick with it. Switching physical therapists in midstream will cause a major disruption in a youngster's rehabilitation training; in some cases bringing the athlete back to square one. So unless the fit with the therapist is just untenable, stay the course and continue to work with the original choice.

Be consistent. Consistency is an essential factor in any progressive strength and conditioning program. Injury rehabilitation is no different. Missing treatment and/or rehab sessions (even periodically) is not an option for the competitive, improvement-conscious young athlete. If the goal after sustaining an injury is to get back to action at full strength as soon as possible, adhering to a consistent rehabilitation schedule is a must. Remember, consistency plus hard work equals a successful rehabilitation.

Patience. Patience will be severely tested when coming back from an injury, particularly for youngsters. They are generally an impatient bunch, especially when they're asked to curtail their physical activity. Like it or not (and most young athletes won't), the body has its own timetable for recovery independent of anyone's opinion about it. It only responds to the proper ration of exercise, treatment, and rest spread over the appropriate period of time. Realizing this need for patience early on in an athletic career will save youngsters much anguish and frustration when it comes to dealing with injuries.

Don't come back too soon. Although most youngsters will no doubt be tempted, coming back to sports action before being physically ready is a major mistake, one that will put young athletes at risk for re-injury—not to mention lackluster performance. The list of high-profile competitors who have returned too soon from injury only to re-injure themselves would fill this book many times over. Regardless of whatever outside pressures youngsters may encounter from coaches, teammates, fans, and family members, they must aspire to keep their own counsel and take all the time they need for recovery and rehabilitation before jumping back into the competitive fray.

Injury rehabilitation never really ends. Once youngsters return to full strength after rehabilitating from an injury, the special attention given to the formerly-injured area is not over. It is imperative that young athletes continue to monitor the region of the body for signs of aggravation and pain. These sensations may be precursors to re-injury and should be dealt with immediately and appropriately (rest, treatment, extra flexibility or strength work, etc.).

Common Youth Sports Injuries

While active, athletic youngsters incur a wide variety of injuries, some (because of the frequency with which they occur) deserve special attention. These injuries are discussed in the following paragraphs.

Rotator Cuff Tendonitis

The muscles of the rotator cuff stabilize the shoulder joint. When athletic performance requires more of these small muscles than the force they are capable of generating, the tendon becomes overinvolved, thus causing pain and inflammation. (Tendons are not designed to absorb as much stress as are muscles.)

Injuries to the rotator cuff region of the shoulder are common among young athletes. They occur most often in activities that require overhead shoulder action such as volleyball, tennis, baseball, swimming, and weightlifting.

The key to preventing (and recovering from) injury to the rotator cuff lies in an aggressive strengthening program, one that incorporates a variety of specialized, low-resistance exercises for the shoulder girdle. While the strength-training section of this book provides rotator cuff exercises, because of the precise nature of strengthening this area, it is strongly suggested that all youngsters, regardless of their experience in the weight room, enlist the help of a physical therapist and/or strength and conditioning specialist when learning rotator strengthening movements.

Lower Leg Stress Fractures

Stress fractures to the lower leg are overuse injuries that occur when too much stress causes the outside of the bone to crack. They are most common in athletes who participate in sports or training activities that entail repetitive impact to the ground, such as long distance runners, basketball players, soccer players, and lacrosse players. These injuries are serious, painful, and, if not treated correctly, potentially chronic.

Since stress fractures tend to develop over many weeks, they can often be recognized and treated before they become serious. Minor pain and irritation in the lower leg, especially when it's near the bone, may very well be a precursor to a full-blown stress fracture. As such, when a youngster complains of pain in the shin region, instead of dismissing it as "shin splints" (the blanket term used in the sports community to describe shin pain), parents should schedule a visit to a sports medicine doctor for diagnosis and treatment. This course of action may save the young athlete many hours of downtime and pain.

Youngsters can also significantly lower their susceptibility to stress fractures by keeping calcium intake reasonably high (1500mg per day for teens), utilizing soft surfaces when engaging in high-impact activities, avoiding overtraining, and by incorporating specially-designed orthotics (arch supports) in their athletic footwear and, if necessary, in their everyday walking shoes. This advice is especially crucial for young female athletes, as they are more susceptible to stress fractures than are their male counterparts.

If a stress fracture to the lower leg does occur, healing time is usually between six and eight weeks, depending upon the severity of the injury and the patient's biology.

During downtime, young athletes should maintain conditioning by engaging in non-impact activities such as swimming, water workouts, and stationary biking.

Elbow Injuries

Elbow injuries are common in sports where throwing is prevalent, such as field events (shot put, javelin), football (quarterbacks), and especially baseball and softball (pitchers). Upper body weightlifting can also aggravate the elbow region. Young athletes are much more susceptible to elbow injuries than are older competitors since their musculatures are not fully developed and their growth plates are not yet closed.

Two major factors are important in the prevention of elbow injuries. First is adhering to a consistent and aggressive strengthening program that pays special attention to forearm and shoulder development. Second involves limiting overuse. For instance, little league baseball provides specific guidelines for how many pitches youngsters should throw in a given week. Following these recommendations (and others like them) is required for all youngsters involved in throwing intensive activities.

Secondary prevention methods include icing the elbow after intense use, throwing with proper mechanics, and visiting a sports medicine doctor at the first sign of elbow pain.

Chronic Lower Back Pain

Many athletes at all levels of sport experience chronic back pain. Youngsters are no exception. This type of pain comes about when a bulging disc is pushing on a nerve, and it is usually recognizable by a shooting pain down through the lower leg, sometimes extending to the toes. Needless to say it can be very debilitating, often causing the athlete to miss long stretches of action.

Strengthening the core region of the body (which includes the muscles of the mid-section, lower back, and hips) and maintaining lower body flexibility (especially in the hamstrings) are the keys to preventing chronic back pain in young athletes. Complete core strengthening and stretching protocols are discussed elsewhere in this book.

Young Women and Knee Injuries

Among young female athletes, the preponderance of serious knee injuries, especially the dreaded anterior cruciate ligament (ACL) tear, is alarming. According to the American Association of Orthopedic Surgeons, female high school and college athletes are as much as seven times more likely to tear their ACLs during competition than are male athletes at the same levels. Even more conservative studies put the ratio at 4:1 girls to boys. There are numerous theories about why this discrepancy occurs. Many in the medical community believe that young women are more susceptible to these types of injuries because of their wider hip structure; looser, weaker, and smaller ligaments; and weaker hamstring muscles in relation to the quadriceps.

Regardless of the reasons, one thing is beyond debate: ACL tears are extremely painful and debilitating. They can keep a young athlete out of action for extended periods of time, and in many instances will contribute to future deterioration of the knee joint. Additionally, once a serious knee injury is sustained, the chances of re-injury to the area increases many-fold.

The best defense against these incapacitating injuries is, as they say, a good offense. A good offense in this case refers to proper and aggressive training. Knee injury prevention programs should include a combination of balance exercises (Chapter 9) and a variety of lower body strengthening movements that focus on the muscles of the hips and the upper legs, with an emphasis on the hamstrings (Chapter 7). Learning and adhering to proper running and landing technique, maintaining an ideal body weight, and improving flexibility will also help curtail the incidence of injuries to the knee.

4

Youth Sports Nutrition

Make sure not to blink while reading this chapter, or you'll be in jeopardy of missing the next diet craze. That's an exaggeration, but not by much. Never a simple subject, nutrition has become downright confusing in this day and age, as diet recommendations seem to change by the hour (if not the minute). Foods that only a few short years ago were considered nutritious, healthy, and energy promoting are now, according to some, to be avoided at all costs. Conversely, food choices labeled the devils of the nutritional world for decades currently stand as the popular darlings of the diet set. Don't get to comfortable with any of it, because these and other opinions about what constitutes sound nutrition can change like the wind, especially when market share (i.e., money) is at stake.

What then is an improvement-conscious young athlete to do in this contentious and ever-changing nutritional environment? The advice is simple and entails just two words, the same two words youth coaches constantly repeat (yell) to their athletes during sports competitions and team practices: stay balanced. Yes, the good ol' balanced diet, consisting of ample complex carbohydrates, reasonable portions of high-quality protein, adequate fat intake, and plenty of hydrating water is still the ticket to high performance in sports. Of course, you will have some variations. For instance, a young 10,000-meter runner will usually require more in the way of complex carbohydrates than will a junior high school third baseman. And a developing football interior lineman trying to add muscular weight to his frame in order to compete at the next level will more than likely consume more grams of protein proportionate to his body weight than would a mid-teenage female high jumper. But on the whole, balance is still the name of the game when it comes to a young athlete's nutritional program.

This chapter will help guide the reader through the minefield that has become sports nutrition, taking into account the specialized needs of the young athlete along the way and ignoring, for the most part, any of the "diet noise" that constantly barrages the senses of Americans on a daily basis. It will include a thorough discussion of the components of balanced nutrition, complete with recommended percentages for each of the basic food groups, and explanations of how vitamins, minerals, and all-important water interact within the body. The controversial topics of nutritional supplementation and performance-enhancing drugs will be covered comprehensively as well, especially with respect to how they affect the youth sports community. Safe strategies for gaining and losing weight and productive ways to encourage youngsters to eat in a healthful and athletic-enhancing manner will also be presented. The chapter concludes with sample meal plans that youngsters, with help from parents and coaches, can implement as part of a year-round dietary program.

Components of Balanced Nutrition

Water

Approximately two-thirds of an individuals body mass is composed of water. It is without question the most important ingredient in any young athlete's diet. Water performs many critical functions in the body, including modulating body temperature (a key factor during vigorous exercise), lubricating joints, carrying nutrients to cells and waste products away from cells, and helping the digestion and absorption of food.

Drinking a minimum of eight 12-ounce glasses of water each day is imperative for young, active athletes. On hot, humid days, or when high amounts of energy are expended, up to twelve 12-ounces glasses should be consumed. Other liquids such as lemonade, various fruit juices, and sports drinks such as Gatorade or Powerade basically have the same effect on the body as water (all are water-based.) However, pure water is still the simplest (and least expensive) way to remain hydrated and is the recommended beverage of choice for youngsters involved in sports and conditioning programs. Alcoholic, caffeinated, and carbonated beverages should be avoided as much as possible, as they include ingredients that actually contribute to dehydration.

Young athletes should aspire to keep their fluid intake high throughout the day, not just before, during, and after athletic competitions or workouts. To accomplish this, it is suggested that youngsters carry a filled water bottle with them at all times, even on days when no sports activities are planned. Remaining optimally hydrated contributes to buoyant health and peak athletic performance. Make sure it's part of a youngster's lifestyle.

Carbohydrates (Percent of total calories = 55 to 60 percent. Calories per gram = 4)

Carbohydrates are the easiest form of food for the body to turn into energy. However, not all are created equal. Complex carbohydrates—which include potatoes, rice, vegetables, beans, breads, and pastas—provide long-term energy and are easily digested. These foods contain necessary nutrients such as B vitamins and will always be the mainstay in a young athlete's nutritional plan. Complex carbohydrates will also be the primary food for pre-competition, pre-practice, and pre-conditioning workout meals.

Simple carbohydrates, such as fruits and processed sugars, while easily digested, provide only short-term energy. With exception of fresh fruit and some fruit juices, which provide excellent sources of important nutrients (minerals, fiber, vitamins), simple carbohydrates should be eaten only in moderation.

How many grams of carbohydrates youngsters consume per day is a function of activity level and individual metabolism. As a rule of thumb, when engaging in intense training, young athletes should multiply their body weight by five to derive the appropriate number of carbohydrate grams to be eaten each day. During light training intervals or inactive periods, three should be used as the multiplier. As mentioned previously, these multipliers are just approximations and much will depend on the individual. However, because most active young athletes have extremely fast metabolisms, it is usually better to err on high side of carbohydrate intake.

Proteins (Percent of total calories = 25 to 30 percent. Calories per gram = 4)

The body utilizes protein to build and repair muscle tissue. Obviously, hard-training young athletes who are engaging regularly in sports (and physically demanding conditioning activities such as weightlifting) must include ample amounts of high quality protein in their diets. The best sources of protein are eggs, fish, red meat, poultry (chicken, turkey, etc.), and dairy products. These foods are considered complete proteins, since they contain all the amino acids necessary to build muscle. Incomplete proteins, such as most plant proteins, lack one or more of the essential amino acids and can only contribute to the muscle building process if consumed in the proper combinations. Food combining—such as eating beans and rice together in the same meal—experienced a good deal of popularity some years back during the low-fat diet craze. However, this practice has proved difficult for many who are not preparing their own food on a regular basis (most of us in today's busy world). For parents who are interested in food combining, many books and websites cover the topic in detail. Unless involved in a weight-gaining program (discussed later in the chapter), eating approximately 0.5 to 0.6 grams of high-quality protein daily per pound of body weight is sufficient for young athletes.

Fats (Percent of total calories = 15 to 20 percent. Calories per gram = 9)

Needed by the body, fats supply a major source of energy, protect vital organs, and help to prevent starvation during times of insufficient food intake. The problem is that the average American youngster, including many competitive young athletes, derives in the neighborhood of 50 percent of his calories from fat. While the once-popular extremely low-fat diet is not suggested here, neither is the fast-food-laden, 50-percent-fat diet. This amount of fat consumption can add unwanted weight to the physique and raise cholesterol levels, which increases the risk of heart disease. To ensure that youngsters keep their fat intake at reasonable levels, parents should make a conscious effort to not overserve fried foods, fatty meats, and high-fat dairy products (ice cream, whole milk, brie cheese, etc.). Instead, try to encourage the consumption of low-fat protein sources, such as egg whites, fresh fish, lean red meats, skim or 1% milk, yogurt, and poultry.

Vitamins

Vitamins perform a variety of important functions in the body. For example, vitamin D assists in the absorption of calcium and vitamin C enhances resistance to infection. While vitamins are not a source of energy, they do release energy from food consumed. In essence, they ensure that calories are utilized appropriately. Vitamins are only needed by the body in small amounts and can, for the most part, be obtained from eating a balanced, nutritionally sound diet.

Minerals

More than 20 mineral elements are found in the body, 17 of which are necessary in a young athlete's diet. Some of the most important include calcium, iron, copper, iodine, magnesium, manganese, phosphorus, potassium, and zinc. Minerals help to build strong bones, maintain bodily tissues, and contribute to muscles working efficiently. Most minerals that the body requires can be obtained by eating conscientiously.

While regular mineral supplementation is not necessary for boys, young girls in Phases 2 and 3 may want to consider supplementing their diets with extra calcium and iron. Calcium helps to prevent osteoporosis, which is much more common in women than in men. Ingesting adequate calcium is especially important during the years of 12 to 16 when bone structure is developing. Active female athletes of menstrual age also need to keep their iron intake reasonably high (about 18 milligrams per day) or risk developing iron deficiency anemia, which has been known to cause performance deficits in competitive athletes.

Nutritional Supplements

The vast array of nutritional supplements available today is mind-boggling. Some promise to build massive amounts of strength and muscle. Others claim to burn fat, making bodies lean and muscularly defined in a few short weeks. Still others, like the popular supplement creatine, are said to improve sports and workout performance.

Regardless of whether the previous claims have merit or not, one thing is beyond dispute: nutritional supplements are big business. Sales are estimated at 50 million dollars annually and growing rapidly from year to year. Young athletes spend many of those dollars looking for that elusive competitive edge. Much of the popularity of supplements among youngsters can be traced to the aggressive marketing efforts by manufactures, which more often than not feature superstar professional athletes as spokesmen. (This marketing strategy seems to be working, as up to 50 percent of high school age athletes admit to using dietary supplements on a semi-regular basis.)

Despite their widespread popularity throughout the sports and fitness communities, the jury is still out concerning how much benefit dietary supplements actually provide. Many experts in the nutritional field feel that if youngsters are eating a well-balanced, nutritionally-sound diet, the need for supplementation is minimal, or even non-existent. In fact, the American Academy of Pediatrics believes that dietary supplements have no place in the meal plans of children. Additionally, since the supplement industry is unregulated (allowing manufactures much leeway in what they actually put on the market), young athletes and those who guide them should approach supplements with extreme caution. The following are some of the most popular dietary supplements:

Protein powders and mega-mass tablets. Manufacturers of protein powders and so-called "muscle building" pills claim that their products allow for protein to be assimilated more efficiently by the body, with the ultimate result being more muscular development. The truth is that protein is protein regardless of its source, and these aggressively promoted potions are more likely to produce stomach cramps than they are to add substantial amounts of lean muscle tissue to a young athlete's frame. Protein requirements for youngsters can and should be met through conventional food sources. While these supplements aren't harmful, they are expensive and best off left on the shelf.

Creatine. Creatine is a natural substance manufactured in the body and serves as a small energy source, assisting in the execution of explosive, short duration athletic activities such as swinging a baseball bat or jumping for a rebound. According to proponents, adding or loading creatine into the system will enhance an athlete's ability to perform dynamic actions. Some also claim that regular creatine supplementation enhances recovery after intense workouts. It must be made clear, however, that creatine supplementation does not actually build muscle tissue; it allows athletes to train harder, with the byproduct being increased muscular development.

Creatine has been researched and studied more than most nutritional supplements; however, many medical professionals still feel that more needs to be learned about its long-term effects. Before engaging in any type of creatine supplementation program, youngsters (along with their parents) should first consult a sports medicine physician.

Sport drinks and energy bars. To the surprise of many, energy bars such as Power Bars and sports drinks such as Gatorade are considered nutritional supplements. Of all the supplements mentioned in this chapter, these two types are the safest and potentially among the most effective. Both are useful for energy maintenance purposes, and sports drinks can provide a great source of hydrating fluids, especially for those young athletes who engage in continuous endurance-type activities (e.g., running or cycling) for an extended period of time (i.e., an hour or longer). Sports drinks can also be appropriate for young athletes who participate in relatively strenuous activities conducted in a high-humidity environment. High in both protein and carbohydrates, energy bars are particularly convenient for busy athletes, since they are small in size, are packaged securely, and have an extremely long shelf life. In reality, many elite athletes consume these products before, during, and after competitions, team practices, and conditioning workouts. Depending upon the circumstances, young athletes might also consider doing the same. It is important to keep in mind, however, that the nutritional impact of a glass of milk and a peanut butter and jelly sandwich is quite comparable to an energy bar and that except in high-humidity conditions and in situations where individuals are engaging in whole-body activities on a non-stop basis for at least an hour, water is more than adequate to meet the fluid-replacement needs of most young athletes.

Androstenedione. Androstenedione (popularly known as Andro) made headlines some years back when it was spotted in the locker of former baseball home run king Mark McGuire by a sports reporter. While recognized as a legal supplement (at least by Major League Baseball at the time), Andro is part of the dangerous and confusing over-the-counter steroid precursors marketed to young athletes. These derivatives are metabo-lized into steroids once they enter the body and thus, according to many in the medical community, produce similarly harmful side effects. Unfortunately, the over-the-counter availability of steroid precursors gives the wrong impression that they're harmless. They're not! As such, this (alleged) supplement should be avoided by all young athletes.

Ephedra. This dangerous product is found in numerous weight-loss formulas. Side effects of ephedra include dizziness, stomach cramps, insomnia, high blood pressure, and seizures. It has been implicated as a contributing factor in the recent death of Baltimore Orioles pitcher Steve Belcher. Ephedra's negative publicity has lead to its removal in many fat-burners, even enticing marketers to claim, usually in big, bright letters, that their products are now "Ephedra Free." Unfortunately, some of the replacement ingredients in these formulas are also proving to be dangerous. Obviously, the use of Ephedra, or any similar product, is not recommended for young athletes.

Glucosamine chondroitin. This supplement has shown to substantially lessen joint soreness, particularly in the knee and shoulder regions, with no apparent harmful side effects. Glucosamine chondroitin has been highly touted in Europe, and is beginning to gain a large following in the United States as well. Consuming this product regularly (especially for those young athletes recovering from joint injury/surgery) is suggested by many in the medical and injury rehabilitation fields. The dosage recommendations vary somewhat, but one to two pills per day containing a combination of 1500 mg. of glucosamine and 1200 mg. of chondroitin is in the range for hard-training young athletes. This supplement is widely available at drug and health food stores.

Steroids and Other Performance-Enhancing Drugs

Notwithstanding the recent wave of attention in the news media, steroids and other so-called "performance-enhancing" drugs have been prevalent in the sports world for many years. Their use has mostly been linked to professional and Olympic athletes, but recent research seems to indicate that the consumption of these dangerous drugs is much more widespread. This new breed of user includes adult fitness enthusiasts, adult recreational athletes, and (most alarmingly) young athletes. Some studies show that up to 10 percent of high school athletes experiment with steroids or other similar drugs at some point in their scholastic sports careers. These estimates may be low, considering the fact that many youngsters are hesitant to admit any type of drug use— be it of the muscle building variety or otherwise.

Taking their cue from superstar athletes, many impressionable youngsters (complete with their indestructible attitudes) believe that partaking in these substances is a win/win proposition: gain muscle size and strength with no harmful side effects. Of course, this line of thinking is erroneous. While steroids and drugs like them may help an athlete build additional muscle mass, strength, and power in the short term, they also produce numerous long-term harmful side effects that can not only ruin athletic careers, but lives as well. Following is a list of many of the most serious side effects of performance enhancing drugs:

- Liver cancer
- High blood pressure
- Increased risk of heart disease
- Impaired immune system
- Stunted growth because of premature closing of growth plates
- Increase in connective tissue (tendons and ligaments) injuries due to the stress of carrying unnatural bulk
- Excessive aggressiveness
- Muscle pulls and tears
- Infertility
- Testicular atrophy

One glance at the list of side effects makes it clear that youth coaches, trainers, and especially parents must do everything in their power to discourage young athletes from even casually experimenting with steroids and other illegal sports performance drugs. The health dangers should be emphasized regularly, and any signs of use (back acne, deeper voice, and dramatic increases in muscular body weight) must be addressed immediately. Parents and coaches may also want to stress to young athletes that if drug tests show positive results for banned substances such as steroids, suspensions, loss of potential scholarships, and dismissal from teams are just some of the potential outcomes.

Ironically, some of the well-documented steroid-related scandals involving high profile athletes may actually help to convince young athletes to stay clear of these synthetic muscle builders. Ramifications of asterisks on records, broken contracts, serious and (in many cases) mysterious illnesses, and lost reputations seem to be opening young eyes to the consequences of steroid/performance-enhancing drug use. But adults involved with young athletes must nevertheless continue to persevere in their quest to keep steroids and other dangerous drugs out of youth sports.

Alcohol, Recreational Drugs, and Tobacco

For serious, hard-training young athletes, staying clear of alcohol, drugs, and tobacco should be obvious. Unfortunately, in our complicated society fraught with hard choices and peer pressure, it is not always so cut and dry. That being said, a few things are certain and can't be debated: using any of the previously mentioned substances, even on a casual basis, can lead to addiction, serious health problems, and a reduction in athletic performance. Numerous well-known athletes from a variety of sports have short-circuited their careers due to alcohol and drug abuse. All youngsters should do themselves and their athletic careers a favor and abstain from alcohol, drugs, and tobacco.

Weight Control

Young athletes have a variety of reasons for wanting to gain or lose weight. Some may aspire to increase physical strength and power in order to perform better in their chosen sport(s), thus requiring additional muscular body weight. Others feel that losing weight will increase their speed, quickness, and endurance, making them more efficient and explosive athletes. In either case, youngsters should take care to work within their genetic make-up (i.e., ectomorph: slim build; mesomorph: muscular build; endomorph: heavy/large build), and aspire to maintain a reasonably low level of body fat.

Calories: How Many for the Young Athlete?

Determining the ideal number of calories for growing, active youngsters is extremely difficult. Formulas for caloric intake vary widely depending on growth, age, physical maturity, activity level, and individual metabolism. Also, the aforementioned factors change constantly, making it virtually impossible to pinpoint the exact calorie requirements for youngsters at any given point in time.

The most efficient way to judge whether a young athlete is consuming enough high-quality food is to monitor weight, growth, and above all, energy level. Doing so, of course, will require some degree of diligence on the part of parents, youth coaches, and family physicians. However, it is a far better approach than trying to follow preconceived, so-called scientific recommendations, which only deal with the "average" child (as if there is such a thing).

Many Young Athletes Don't Eat Enough

A large number of young athletes, especially young female athletes, don't eat enough. With all the talk of youth obesity currently circulating throughout the news media, this may come as a surprise to some, but focused studies seem to confirm it.

Calorie expenditure by youngsters during athletic activities (participating in various sports, engaging in strength and conditioning training, working on developing skills, etc.) is also underestimated, sometimes by as much as 25 percent or more. In fact, recent research has shown that among the majority of young sports competitors, energy intake (food consumption) appeared to be lower than energy expenditure. Even a more alarming aspect of this research is that a large percentage of young female team sport athletes were found to be trying to lose weight unnecessarily during their competitive seasons. Significant weight loss over the course of a competitive sports season will usually lead to decreases in performance.

It must be clearly understood by anyone involved in youth sports that the overwhelming majority of dedicated young athletes are extremely active on a year-round basis. Combine this with the fact that their bodies are growing rapidly, and the need for substantial calories is exceedingly necessary.

Weight Gain

In order to gain weight in a safe and efficient manner, young athletes should focus on two factors. First, more high-quality calories (short on junk food, long on lean protein and complex carbohydrates) must be taken in than expended. And second, a year-round strength training program which focuses on building maximum amounts of muscle mass should be undertaken. This approach will ensure that the additional weight comes in the form of lean muscle tissue and not unwanted, performance inhibiting fat.

Youngsters and those who guide them should always keep in mind that being in a weight-gaining mode doesn't mean eating anything and everything in one's path. Fat consumption should still remain moderate, and overindulging in starchy carbohydrates is strongly discouraged. Small amounts of additional muscle-building protein can and should be added to a youngsters diet during a weight-gaining cycle. Limits do exist, however. The body can only metabolize (use) 20 to 30 grams of protein in any given three- to four-hour time period. As such, the best way to maximize protein intake is to incorporate five or six small, protein rich meals spread equally throughout the day.

Weight Loss

For young athletes wishing to lose weight, the first point of emphasis is that the scale should never be the ultimate judge. As mentioned previously, every individual youngster has a unique build, and actual weight is not nearly as important as body composition (relative amounts of muscle, bone, and fat in the body). Overweight youngsters should always make losing body fat and gaining lean muscle tissue their priority. Since muscle weighs more than fat, what a young athlete weighs is far less important than how it is distributed throughout the body. The majority of top-level athletes would be considered overweight by American medical body weight charts. As such, these charts mean nothing to competitive young athletes and should be ignored.

Numerous strategies can be implemented to lose weight and improve body composition ratios. Some of the most time-tested strategies are as follows:
- Eat five to six smaller meals per day as opposed to the traditional three larger ones.
- Avoid eating heavy, calorie-laden foods late at night before retiring.
- Eat high-fiber, reasonably low-fat meals regularly.
- Moderate intake of starchy carbohydrates (such as whipped potatoes, non-whole wheat pastas, and white breads).
- Get the majority of protein from low-fat sources (such as fish, lean meats, egg whites, poultry, and skim milk).
- Avoid fried foods.
- Keep away from empty calories (calories without any nutritional value) such as soft drinks and sugary snacks.
- Drink ample amounts of fresh water in order to flush the system.
- Engage in some form of regular aerobic exercise. (See Chapter 5 for aerobic training options and parameters.)
- Strength train consistently. Building lean muscle tissue will help youngsters burn fat more efficiently.
- Stay clear of fad diets and diet pills/potions. These never work in the long run and often cause health problems.

Meals for Competitions and Workouts

Pre-Competition/Workout Meal

Not so long ago, pre-competition meals for athletes usually consisted of a 12-ounce, well-done steak, or some other high-fat meat, a baked potato, piled high with butter and/or sour cream, and a small serving of some type of vegetable. Eating a high-protein, high-fat pre-competition meal was a tradition that stood for decades in sports circles.

Finally, after years of research (and numerous complaints of stomach cramps from athletes), the sports nutrition community has come to its senses. They've learned that fatty, protein rich foods are difficult to digest, thus causing energy depletion in the body, stomach discomfort, and lethargy—not exactly what athletes are looking for prior to a competition, team practice, or conditioning workout.

A pre-competition or pre-workout meal for young athletes should always include ample portions of complex carbohydrates, very little protein and fat, and large amounts of hydrating liquids. As mentioned earlier in this chapter, complex carbohydrates such as pastas, pancakes, and rice are easily digested and, when broken down in the body, produce glucose, which supplies the body's energy needs. Before intense exertion (such as a conditioning workout, basketball game, or soccer match) having large amounts of energy available is obviously crucial to success.

Pre-competition and pre-workout meals should be planned three to three-and-a-half hours before the scheduled activity. However, since metabolism speed in youngsters vary, individual needs should be taken into consideration when establishing pre-activity meal times. For instance, some young athletes may, in addition to their pre-competition/workout meal, require a small, easily digestible snack such as an energy bar or a few rice cakes within an hour or so of a competition or workout to perform at their best. While others, because of their slower digestive systems, are best served pushing the pre-competition/workout meal out to four hours before scheduled high-intensify exertion.

Snacks During Competition/Workouts

Anyone who even casually follows golf on television has seen Tiger Woods munching on a banana or energy bar at some point during his eighteen-hole walk. This activity is no coincidence. Not only is Mr. Woods perhaps the most talented golfer ever to swing a club, but also among the most intelligent and conscientious when it comes to nutrition. Maintaining energy by light snacking during breaks in competition is highly recommended for all young athletes who engage in time consuming sporting events such as tennis matches, football games, or decathlon competitions. This strategy, which should be implemented during long workouts as well, will help to keep glycogen stores high, allowing concentration to remain sharp and physical capabilities steady. Some of the best sources of in-competition snack foods include fresh fruit, sports drinks, energy bars, and graham crackers.

Post-Competition/Post-Workout Eating

Eating after a hard-fought sports competition or an energy-draining conditioning session is a two-fold endeavor. First, 15 to 20 minutes after physical activity concludes, eating a combination protein/carbohydrate snack such as a banana spread lightly with peanut butter or a medium-sized container of yogurt is suggested. Doing so will help replenish glycogen stores in the muscles and enable youngsters to begin the important physical recovery process immediately and efficiently. Keep in mind, however, that many young athletes, especially those who've just participated in an endurance event or workout, may not be hungry (aerobic training tends to suppress the appetite for a time after exercise). Notwithstanding lack of hunger, the "recovery snack" should under no circumstances be neglected. No exceptions.

Second, approximately two hours after the aforementioned "recovery snack," a normal, well-balanced meal similar to those detailed at the end of the chapter should be consumed. While the "recovery snack" is an important part of the recovery process, it should never take the place of a solid, nutritionally sound post-competition/workout meal. No exceptions here as well.

Tips and Strategies to Help Youngsters Eat Better

Parents should stay involved. While youth coaches, trainers, and program directors can regularly encourage young athletes to eat in a healthy manner, parents are on the front line when it comes to a youngster's food choices. They will be the ones preparing the home-cooked meals, packing the brown bag lunches, stocking the refrigerators, and deciding which restaurants to patronize. It therefore goes without saying that parents will and should take an extremely active role in their child's eating habits.

Learn a youngster's food tastes. Sports nutrition can be a somewhat perplexing topic. One thing about it, however, is for sure: regardless of how healthy or energy promoting a food choice is, if a young athlete doesn't like the taste, all the prodding in the world won't get him to eat it. As such, meal plans should always be developed in tune with a youngster's food tastes. The good news here is that most children are partial to a variety of healthy foods. Building meals around such foods is highly recommended.

Strongly emphasize the connection between sound nutrition and high performance. All dedicated young athletes aspire to perform at their best. In fact, success in the sports arena may very well be their priority in life during this time. Youth coaches, fitness trainers, program directors, and parents should constantly remind youngsters that adhering to healthy eating principles is one of the most important (and controllable) factors related to athletic success. Once this diet/performance connection is established in a young person's mind, conscientious eating will more often than not be the result.

Keep healthy foods around. In addition to preparing healthy meals for breakfast, lunch, and dinner, parents should try to make nutritious foods easily accessible around the house. For instance, put together plates and/or bowls of carrot sticks, pineapple slices, nuts, and whole wheat crackers and place them at convenient locations in the kitchen, den, living room, and so on. Most youngsters, especially rushed teenagers, will grab whatever is in front of them for a snack. So why not make the choices as healthy as possible?

Get them interested. Similar to most large subjects, nutrition can be very interesting. Getting youngsters interested and involved in what they put in their mouths is perhaps the best way of ensuring that a sound nutritional program is maintained over the long term. Individuals who work regularly with young athletes, and especially parents should do all they can to peek this interest in diet. Pick up some simple, easy-to-read sports nutrition books and place them conveniently around the house or workout area, find out what a youngster's favorite athlete eats regularly (as long as it's healthy, that is) and post a corresponding meal plan on the refrigerator or gym bulletin board, and of course, continue to emphasize the health, performance, and cosmetic benefits of adhering to a proper diet. Igniting curiosity in nutrition will pay great dividends throughout a youngster's athletic career and life.

Periodic junk food snacks are okay. Trying to impose a Spartan diet routine on a youngster is an impossible task, one that is more likely to short circuit a sound nutritional program than it is to engender healthy eating habits. Periodic treats such as cookies, candy bars, and ice cream cones are fine for active young athletes as long as they are consumed infrequently and not used as meal replacements. These "diet breaks" may actually contribute toward youngsters eating better over the long term.

Sample Meal Plans for Young Athletes

Tables 4-1 through 4-5 detail sample meal plans for young athletes. The suggestions are meant to be a basic guide only. What diet plan a youngster ultimately follows will depend on numerous factors, including, but not limited to, food tastes, age, metabolism speed, individual goals, activity level, and health variables.

- Three-quarter cup of oatmeal with sliced half banana and three ounces of 1% milk

- Four medium-sized whole wheat pancakes with maple syrup

- 12-ounce glass of orange juice

- 12-ounce glass of water

Table 4-1. Sample pre-competition meal (afternoon competition)

- Large bowl of whole wheat pasta (approximately five ounces) with marinara sauce

- Large mixed salad with low-fat dressing

- Half a banana with peanut butter

- 12-ounce glass of Gatorade

- 12-ounce glass of water

Table 4-2. Sample pre-competition meal (night competition)

Breakfast:	Three-egg (two yolks) western omelet
	Two slices of dry whole wheat or whole grain bread
	One-half cup bowl of oatmeal with raisins and three ounces of 2% milk
	12-ounce glass of grapefruit juice
	12-ounce glass of water
Lunch:	Large turkey sandwich on rye bread with lettuce, tomato and mustard
	Medium-sized bowl of vegetable soup
	Two 12-ounce glasses of water
Mid-Afternoon Snack:	Five whole wheat crackers spread with peanut butter
	12-ounce glass of apple juice
Dinner:	Large piece of grilled fish (salmon, tuna, halibut, or swordfish)
	Baked potato with low-fat sour cream
	Medium mixed salad with Italian dressing
	Small slice of pound cake
	Two 12-ounce glasses of water

Table 4-3. Sample daily meal plan for young athletes

Breakfast:	Two poached eggs on one large slice of whole wheat or whole grain bread
	Medium-sized bowl of cold cereal (Cheerios, Total, or Special K) with 1% milk
	12-ounce glass of grape juice
	12-ounce glass of water
Lunch:	Large chef salad with Italian dressing
	Medium-sized whole wheat roll (dry)
	Two 12-ounce glasses of water
Dinner:	12-ounce cut of lean beef
	Small servings of broccoli and cauliflower
	3-ounce bowl of whole wheat pasta with olive oil dressing
	Two 12-ounce glasses of water
P.M. Snack:	One slice of pound cake with strawberries
	12-ounce glass of 2% milk

Table 4-4. Sample daily meal plan for young athletes

Breakfast:	Four scrambled eggs (two yolks) with two slices of pumpernickel toast
	One-half cup of oatmeal with two tablespoons of wheat germ
	12-ounce glass of orange juice
	12-ounce glass of water
Lunch:	Two medium-sized chicken breasts
	One-cup serving of brown rice
	Medium serving of grilled vegetables
	Two 12-ounce glasses of water
Mid-Afternoon Snack:	Medium serving of mixed nuts with dried fruit
	12-ounce glass of water
Dinner:	6-ounce bowl of whole wheat pasta with shrimp topped with marinara sauce
	Medium-sized mixed salad topped with hard cheese slices and Italian dressing
	Small container of low-fat yogurt
	Two 12-ounce glasses of water

Table 4-5. Sample daily meal plan for young athletes

5

Youth Sports Conditioning

In order for youngsters to reach their full potential as athletes, they must be highly conditioned. Attaining peak physical conditioning levels is not only a prerequisite for optimum performance on the playing field, court, or track, but doing so allows young athletes to garner the most out of their improvement workouts whether they be related to skill or conditioning.

Before age-specific conditioning protocols are reviewed, it is important that readers have at least a fundamental understanding of the body's energy systems and the basics of both aerobic and anaerobic conditioning. These topics are discussed in detail in the following sections.

Energy Systems

The energy released from the food a young athlete consumes is utilized to manufacture a chemical compound called adenosine triphosphate, or ATP. Muscle action is powered by the energy yielded from the hydrolysis of this compound. ATP can be produced by three pathways—two are considered anaerobic (without oxygen), the other aerobic (with oxygen).

The first pathway is called ATP-PC (phosphocreatine). PC, similar to ATP, is stored in the muscle and has an extremely high-energy yield. The PC system itself is anaerobic, and the total amount of ATP that can be produced through this mechanism is finite. The ATP-PC pathway becomes involved when muscles are giving maximal effort, such as jumping as high as possible, performing a maximum weight lift, or sprinting 15 yards. The energy reserves from this system only lasts approximately five to 15 seconds.

The second pathway capable of producing ATP is anaerobic glycolysis—frequently referred to as the lactic acid system. This system, as the name suggests, is anaerobic and does not involve oxygen. During glycolysis, carbohydrates (glycogen or glucose) are broken down to form ATP. Anaerobic glycolysis takes over where the ATP-PC system leaves off, allowing youngsters to extend high-intensity exercise. However, the buildup of lactic acid (lactate) will trigger fatigue (and the slowing of anaerobic glycolysis) even in the most highly conditioned athletes within two-and-a-half minutes or so after the start of rigorous work. In essence, the process forces the athlete to discontinue exercising, or at least lower the intensity considerably to facilitate the removal of lactic acid from the body. Examples that would bring this system into play include sprinting 400 meters or jumping rope at full speed for two minutes.

The final pathway in the energy production chain is the aerobic system. This system supplies the body with long-term energy and involves the use of oxygen. After two-and-a-half to three minutes of exercise, the body's ATP requirements are met mostly by the aerobic system. Unlike glycolysis, which can only use carbohydrates to free energy, the aerobic metabolism is able to break down both fats and proteins along with carbohydrates to produce ATP. Some popular forms of aerobic exercise include long-distance running, biking, and swimming.

It is important to note that the transition between energy pathways during exercise is not an instantaneous change, but instead a gradual shift from one system to another. For example, when jumping rope with a heavy-corded jump rope for 35 seconds, energy comes from a combination of the ATP-PC system and the lactic acid system. In another example, the energy for running 800 meters as fast as possible would come from both anaerobic pathways and the aerobic system. Table 5-1 gives an example of the energy pathway continuum.

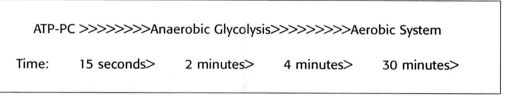

Table 5-1. Energy pathway continuum

Aerobic Conditioning

Aerobic training is usually defined as any reasonably low-intensity activity that is sustained for an extended period of time. Although some fitness professionals feel that aerobic benefits can be achieved in as little as 12 continuous minutes of exercise, for young athletes it is best to work within 20-minute to 60-minute time parameters.

In addition to workout duration, the intensity at which a young athlete exercises must be taken into account. Most experts agree that to acquire satisfactory aerobic benefits, youngsters should exercise somewhere between 70 and 85 percent of their maximal heart rate (max HR). The max HR can be easily figured by subtracting a youngster's age from 220. A 14 year-old athlete, for example, would have a max HR of 206 (220-14= 206). Therefore, in order for that same 14 year-old youngster to incur satisfactory aerobic benefits he would need to elevate his heart rate to between 144 and 175 beats per minute (bpm) during exercise.

A youngster's heart rate can be conveniently calculated by using a heart rate monitor. These devices are easy to use and can be purchased at a fairly nominal cost at most sporting goods stores or from a variety of mail order fitness catalogs. Some state-of-the-art fitness equipment even provide built-in heart rate monitors. If a heart rate monitor is not available, the heart rate can be determined by simply checking the pulse rate by pinpointing the radial artery in the wrist and counting the bpm.

Importance of Developing an Aerobic Base

All athletes, regardless of age, sport, or fitness goals should establish an aerobic base of conditioning. The most important reasons for this are as follows.

General health benefits. While this book is designed for the competitive young athlete, the general health benefits of regular aerobic exercise can't be ignored. Achieving a high level of aerobic fitness is one of the foundations of good health. Engaging in it regularly will help to lower blood pressure, increase HDL cholesterol (the good cholesterol that assists in preventing heart disease), lower the risk of some cancers, and improve cardio-respiratory function. Additionally, those young athletes who make aerobic training part of their sports conditioning regime tend to continue this healthy habit for a lifetime.

Prepares the body for intense activity. Before young athletes engage in any form of high-intensity anaerobic training (interval sprint work, plyometrics, agility/quickness drills, etc.) or participate in competitive movement-oriented sports such as basketball, soccer, or volleyball, it is imperative that they first achieve a solid aerobic base of conditioning. In essence, aerobic training sets the stage for more physically taxing anaerobic activities. Those youngsters who attempt to jump right into anaerobic workouts or competitive situations without preconditioning their aerobic systems are setting themselves up for sports failure, not to mention injury. A minimum of six to eight weeks of aerobic training should precede all sports seasons or intensive anaerobic conditioning workouts.

Improves recovery time. Establishing an aerobic base will greatly enhance a young athlete's ability to recover from intense exertion. Doing so is especially important in sports that involve numerous starts and stops such as football, hockey, tennis, and basketball. For example, after a long, hard-fought point in tennis, an athlete may have 30 seconds or so to rest before beginning the subsequent point. During that half-minute, aerobically fit players will recover sufficiently and be ready to go all-out when the next point starts. On the other hand, less-conditioned individuals will still be feeling the effects of the prior rally as the next point commences. Guess who has the best chance to win the point, not to mention the match?

The benefits of being able to recover quickly are not limited to improving performance in sports competitions. Strength, agility/quickness, plyometric, and speed workouts will be similarly improved. Achieving a solid aerobic base will also enhance a youngster's ability to recover between workouts, allowing them to perform at their physical best day after day.

Weight control. Aerobic exercise speeds up the metabolism significantly, turning the body into a virtual fat-burning furnace. For those youngsters who tend to put on unwanted weight (unfortunately, an all too common problem in this day and age), developing an aerobic base will not only improve their sports and workout performance, but help them shed the pounds as well. Of course, following a sensible, reasonably low-calorie diet plan is also a major component in weight loss.

Maintain condition during down time. Over the course of a young athlete's sports career, engaging in high-intensity sports or conditioning activities will be impossible at times because of injury, lack of playing time, or other unforeseen circumstances. Possessing a well-developed aerobic base will help young athletes maintain their conditioning for longer periods of time, thus speeding their return to more demanding physical efforts.

Anaerobic Conditioning

Physical activity is considered anaerobic when an individual is exercising at about 85 to 100 percent of his maximum heart rate. The following instances are examples when young athletes work anaerobically during sports competition: sprinting the length of a soccer field in pursuit of a dribbling opponent, pitching a fastball in baseball or softball, spiking a volleyball, and playing full-court pressure defense in basketball.

The key to successful anaerobic workouts is intensity. Youngsters must work as hard as they are physically capable for the prescribed time and/or distance. (Please note: physical capabilities for anaerobic training will vary widely between Phases 1, 2, and 3.) As discussed previously, the high-effort nature of anaerobic training allows for only short bouts of exercise, approximately two-and-a-half minutes being the maximum, before fatigue gets the best of even the most soundly conditioned young athlete.

Most anaerobic training programs for youth sports will cover 12 to 18 off-season weeks, depending on level of athlete and sport. The workouts themselves will take place on two non-consecutive days per week. Anaerobic training should only commence after a solid aerobic base of conditioning is achieved. Engaging in high-intensity anaerobic workouts without the proper preconditioning will hinder performance and often leads to injury.

Direct anaerobic training sessions can be continued on a limited basis during competitive sports seasons; however, youth coaches must take into account each youngster's weekly physical activity levels. For example, softball players maybe able to handle two anaerobic workouts per week during the season, since softball game play requires very little in the way of sustained movement. On the other hand, basketball players receive more than enough anaerobic work by participating in their sport, so separate anaerobic workouts would not be necessary during the competitive campaign for most.

Work:Rest Ratios

When designing anaerobic conditioning programs for youth sports, it is critical that specific work:rest ratios be incorporated. The work:rest ratio denotes the work or exercise period of an activity relative to the rest interval. For example, if a youngster sprints for 20 seconds and rests for 40 seconds before sprinting again, the work:rest ratio would be 1:2.

Typically, the longer the bout of anaerobic activity, the more equal the work:rest ratio will be. For instance, going all-out jumping rope for two minutes requires approximately a work:rest ratio of 1:1. While performing an agility drill at full speed for 15 seconds would call for somewhere between a 1:2 to 1:3 work:rest ratio. Keep in mind, work:rest ratios will vary, sometimes significantly, depending upon the conditioning and physical capabilities of the young athlete involved. Youth coaches, program directors, and trainers should remain acutely aware of this when putting young athletes through anaerobic workouts. With young, developing athletes, especially Phase 1 and 2 youngsters, it is always better to err on the side of caution and extend rest periods rather than push them to resume activity too quickly. Table 5-2 summarizes the various durations for anaerobic training and the appropriate work:rest ratios involved.

Work/Time in Seconds	Work:Rest Ratios
0 to 45	1:3
45 to 120	1:2 to 1:1
120 to 150	1:1

Table 5-2. Anaerobic exercise times and approximate work:rest ratios

Popular Forms of Conditioning

Running

Running will be the conditioning option of choice for most young athletes. This choice certainly stands to reason, since the large majority of youth sports—from field hockey to cross-country—require participants to run from place to place during competition. Running also provides perhaps the most efficient of all cardiovascular workouts.

Two other positive byproducts of running are cost (low) and psychological effects (high). Unless a treadmill is purchased for the home, all a young runner need buy is a sturdy pair of running shoes; no fancy equipment or expensive gym membership is required. And nothing in the fitness-training universe clears the head better than a run along a scenic beach or jogging path. Getting out to run is especially helpful to the state of mind of young athletes such as basketball players, volleyball players, and wrestlers who have been cooped up indoors during their long seasons.

Running, as is the case with all exercise modalities, is not without its drawbacks. Most notably it tends to be hard on the knees, feet, shins, and lower back. This stress can be alleviated to some extent by making sure that youngsters take the majority of their running workouts on soft surfaces such as rubberized running tracks, turf fields, or low-cut grass. Treadmills provide a soft pad on which to run; however, working out on them (while effective) is not as beneficial from an athletic standpoint as is moving on solid ground. Young athletes can also lower their chances of incurring a running-related injury by keeping their running shoes up to date. Many running experts suggest maintaining two or even three pairs of running footwear at all times, rotating them every third workout or so. When they show any signs of wearing out, replacing them immediately is recommended. This approach may get somewhat expensive, but it will be well worth the price in terms of preventing injury.

Swimming

Regardless of a young athlete's proficiency as a swimmer, hitting the pool for a training session provides many conditioning benefits. Swimming furnishes a fantastic full-body workout, provides both aerobic and anaerobic benefits, and contributes to the loosening and toning the muscles of the upper body to a high degree. And perhaps the best news of all concerning swimming and water training is that it is extremely easy on the joints and the body in general, offering perhaps the ultimate low-impact workout

If a youngster's swimming skills leave something to be desired, productive water workouts are still possible. A plethora of accessories are available—from kickboards to specially designed flotation vests—to help keep a young athlete's head above water during exercise sessions.

Rowing

World-class rowers are known for their high levels of physical conditioning. They consistently score extremely well in all varieties of cardiovascular fitness tests, and their training regimes are viewed by many in the sports conditioning community as the most demanding in all of competitive athletics.

For most young athletes, rowing workouts will be accomplished indoors on a rowing machine. While rowing on a lake or river is extremely pleasant and exhilarating, it does require some degree of expertise that most youngsters just don't possess. However, if an appropriate body of water is convenient, and the youngster is willing to put in the requisite time to learn, outdoor water rowing is certainly encouraged.

Performed indoors on a rowing machine or outdoors in a single scull, rowing is an extraordinary form of exercises, one that will train both the aerobic and anaerobic metabolisms to the max, while simultaneously building up the muscles of the back, shoulders, biceps, and forearms. Rowing is also fairly easy on the body, as there is no dynamic impact on the joints.

The two standard types of rowing machines are flywheel and hydraulic cylinder rowers. Both machines are adequate; however, most fitness professionals and experienced rowers prefer the flywheel model because it more closely simulates water rowing and places slightly less stress on the lower back region.

Elliptical/Cross Training

The basic idea behind the development of the elliptical/cross trainer was to simulate the running motion minus the foot-fall-related pounding. To a large extent, the machine developers succeeded. More so than any fitness equipment available today, the elliptical/cross trainer does in fact mimic running. In addition, it allows the exerciser to work both the upper and lower body in unison, thus promoting a high level, conditioning workout with an upper body, strength-building component. Unlike many upper/lower body action machines (i.e., cross country ski machines), the elliptical/cross trainer is also easy to operate.

Elliptical/cross trainers are extremely popular and well represented at commercial health and fitness clubs. These machines are available for the home but tend to be somewhat pricy, not to mention cumbersome. All things being considered, these apparatuses rate highly when compared to most fitness conditioning equipment. Be aware, however, that while elliptical/cross trainers do simulate running to a large extent, they should not be used as a full-time replacement for running. Running is the suggested conditioning vehicle for most competitive young athletes and should be employed for the lion's share of conditioning training workouts.

Stationary Cycling

Stationary cycling has long been a staple in fitness circles. For sports training purposes, it has usually been employed in a warm-up and/or cool-down capacity. However, in recent years, with the advent of creative bike-training methods such as spinning (an interval stationary cycling workout), indoor bike work has become popular and useful as a conditioning technique as well. Stationary cycling is especially well suited for youngsters, as it provides a solid low-impact conditioning workout where training intensity can be easily monitored and very little in the way of expertise is required.

The key factor to successful stationary cycling workouts lies in sustaining target heart rate. Where running and swimming, for instance, tend to elevate the heart rate to appropriate levels without much conscious thought or effort, stationary cycling requires full concentration in order to maintain a desired heart rate. Because of this, youngsters are discouraged from either reading or watching television during cycling sessions (listening to music is okay). These activities, while pleasant and time passing, tend to take attention away from the task at hand, which is, of course, garnering the most productive conditioning workout possible.

Numerous types of stationary cycles are available for a young athlete's use. They run the gamut from fancy, computerized models that gauge just about everything (i.e., heart rate, calories burned, revolutions per minute, miles traveled, etc.) to the recumbent variety, where the pedals are positioned straight in front of the rider rather than directly below him, to the simple hand-operated original gathering dust in the family basement or garage. All styles can be utilized effectively as long as the seat is comfortable and adjustable, the pedals durable, and the calibrated tension smooth and operable.

Body Conditioning Classes

Body conditioning classes include a series of functional movements (jumping, hoping, sliding, etc.) performed in a manner that maintains an elevated heart rate. Youngsters favor these workouts because they provide constant and diverse motion, thus minimizing boredom. The classes themselves usually run for about an hour and are offered at most large health clubs and fitness centers. However, these types of workouts can be performed any place where there is ample room and proper terrain (school gym, football field, school yard, etc.). As such, enterprising program coordinators are encouraged to devise their own body conditioning classes, focusing on variety and age-/ability-appropriate training protocols.

Stair Climbing

Once on the cutting edge of the fitness boom, stair climbing fell out of favor with the health club set a decade or so ago. However, in recent years as the equipment has improved, working out on stair climbers is back in vogue—especially in the sports conditioning community. Machine stair climbing basically simulates conventional stair ascending without the inherent impact; feet remain in contact with the pads throughout. While engaging in anaerobic interval training is possible on a stair-climbing machine, the equipment is much more conducive to low and medium intensity aerobic training.

In order for young athletes to get the most out of their stair-climbing workouts, incorporating proper technique is essential. Many trainers make the mistake of using the handlebars for support during execution, either by grabbing them with their hands or leaning over them and bracing themselves on the elbows. Both actions undermine the effectiveness and intensity of the exercise. As such, youngsters should make sure when training on a stair climber to only use the handlebars to maintain balance and pace and not to support their body weight.

Although the newer versions of the stair climbing machine are designed much better than their low-tech brethren of the past, some trainers still complain of knee and hip pain after climbing workouts. This pain is due to the slight hyper-extension of the knee joint during the bottom phase of the movement, along with the repetitive hip motion. Young athletes and those who work with them should monitor this, and if post-workout pain occurs regularly, stair climbing should be discontinued as a conditioning option.

Cross Country Skiing

Cross country skiing provides a phenomenal overall conditioning workout, one that places negligible stress on the knees and lower back and affords the benefit of exercising the upper and lower body in unison. Elite Nordic skiers rate with world-class rowers and Tour De France cyclists when it comes to cardiovascular capacity, and their training regimens are among the most grueling in all of sport.

Unless they live in the vicinity of open snow covered terrain, young athletes will take their cross country skiing workouts on a machine, the most popular of which is the Nordic Track. This apparatus simulates cross country skiing to a surprisingly large degree (case in point, most high-level cross country skiers spend hours upon hours on the Nordic Track, or some other variation in their training) and has been popular in the general fitness community for many years. The only drawback to the Nordic Track (other than the cost, if bought for home use) is that it takes some getting used to, especially if the youngster has no experience on skis. After a few sessions, however, most athletically-oriented young athletes seem to pick it up and are well on their way to productive cross country skiing workouts. Most health clubs, fitness centers, and many school workout facilities have some variation of a cross country ski machine available for use. Table 5-3 illustrates aerobic and anaerobic percentages for specific sports.

	Aerobic %	Anaerobic %
Soccer	40	60
Basketball	25	75
Volleyball	15	85
Field Hockey	30	70
Cross Country	90	10
Football	5	95
Triathlon	95	5
Lacrosse	35	65
Softball	5	95
Boxing	50	50
Field Events	5	95
Distance Swimming	95	5
100-Meter Dash	5	95
Team Handball	25	75
Tennis	30	70

Table 5-3. Aerobic/anaerobic sport-specific percentages

Phase-Specific Conditioning

Phase 1 Conditioning

Conditioning training should be introduced carefully and gradually to Phase 1 children. Because their cardiovascular systems are underdeveloped, capacity to handle heat stress is limited and ability to tolerate the build-up of lactic acid is poor. As such, this age group will concentrate their conditioning workouts on short bursts of speed (i.e., 40-meter dash) and slow and steady-paced, long duration (30 to 35 minutes) activity. Lactic acid system training such as 400 meter sprints are discouraged for Phase 1 athletes.

As is always the case for Phase 1 youngsters, keeping them engaged and interested is a worthy challenge, one that must be met if a fitness program is to be successful. The need for engagement is especially true when it comes to conditioning workouts that can be tedious and somewhat boring for even the most dedicated and patient of adult athletes. Incorporating relay races and obstacle course runs, as well as sports- and game-related activities, as much as possible is strongly suggested for Phase 1 conditioning workouts.

For longer duration conditioning training, program directors may want to try something like this. Locate a two to three mile hiking trail or running course and incorporate five to eight equidistant stations within the course/trail where youngsters are required to do sets of push-ups, crunches, step-ups, body-weight squats, jumping jacks, and so forth. This type of conditioning training is much more mentally tolerable for young children than is swimming repetitive laps in a pool, spending 30 minutes on a stationary bike, or jogging numerous times around a running track. Table 5-4 illustrates examples of proper conditioning protocols for Phase 1 athletes.

Types of Training	Duration/Distance	Speed/Intensity	Sets
Slow, continuous aerobic activity	35 minutes	Low	1
Relay races	40-meter course	Medium	4
Obstacle course	60 meter course	Medium	4
Station course	2.5 miles	Low	1

Table 5-4. Conditioning protocols for Phase 1 athletes

Phase 2 Conditioning

Phase 2 youngsters, along with engaging in brief, all-out bouts of exercise and long duration, even-paced conditioning activities as they did in Phase 1, can begin to train their anaerobic lactic acid systems, albeit in moderation. As mentioned earlier, the lactic acid system picks up where the ATP-PC system leaves off, somewhere between 10 to 15 seconds after the commencement of high-intensity exercise, and remains the dominant energy system over the next minute-and-a-half or so until the aerobic metabolism becomes more involved.

This age group's tolerance for lactic acid build-up is much improved from Phase 1, but it is important to note that it is far from fully developed. As such, while it's appropriate for Phase 2 athletes to participate in 200- to 500-meter runs, the intensity should be tempered. In other words, pushing through at full speed is neither necessary nor suggested. Running distances of less than 150 meters or exercise engaged in for 25 seconds or less can be performed at full throttle by this age group.

Making conditioning activities fun is still important during Phase 2; however, youngsters of this age group should now have the patience and discipline to handle less-exciting forms of conditioning such as long distance jogging, biking, and swimming. Youth coaches, trainers, program directors, and parents should be aware that Phase 2 athletes are susceptible to a wide variety of overuse/repetitive impact-related injuries. This tendency is especially true for those youngsters experiencing rapid spurts in growth. Female athletes also seem to sustain more of these types of injuries during this phase than do their male counterparts. To lower the incidence of overuse/repetitive impact injuries, youngsters should avoid running/jogging/jumping on hard surfaces, and aspire to maintain a balanced approach to conditioning, which includes liberal use of low-impact activities (biking, stair climbing, rowing, swimming, etc.). Table 5-5 illustrates examples of proper conditioning protocols for Phase 2 athletes.

Types of Training	Duration/Distance	Speed/Intensity	Sets
Uphill sprints	30 meters	High	4 to 6
Slow, continuous aerobic activity	30 to 40 minutes	Low	1
Interval sprints	200 to 300 meters	Medium	3 to 4
Rope jumping	1.5 minutes	Medium	2 to 4

Table 5-5. Conditioning Protocols for Phase 2 athletes

Phase 3 Conditioning

All energy systems can be fully trained at this stage of a young athlete's development. The ability to tolerate lactic acid, brought about by a combination of prior training in Phases 1 and 2 and the natural physical maturation process, is improving rapidly for Phase 3 youngsters. High-intensity training such as repetitive 200- to 400-meter interval sprints can now be regularly incorporated into conditioning workouts. Aerobic systems are also becoming highly developed, allowing Phase 3 athletes to sustain conditioning activities for longer periods of time without tiring.

Perhaps the biggest difference between Phase 3 conditioning training and the prior two phases (other than the intensity of the workouts, of course) is the shift toward sport-specific training protocols. Diversity in conditioning is minimized (but still present) in Phase 3, as improving sports performance takes precedence. For example, athletes whose priority sport is basketball will continue to incorporate aerobic training sessions in their conditioning program; however, this type of work will only take place in the early off-season months. After that, anaerobic, basketball-specific workouts will be performed exclusively. (Please note: once an aerobic base is established, it can be maintained through regular anaerobic exercise.)

At the other end of the conditioning spectrum would be cross country runners. These young athletes will give the majority of their conditioning training time to aerobic workouts both in and out of season, with just periodic speed (anaerobic) sessions incorporated as needed throughout the year. Other sports such as boxing and soccer are examples of activities that require a more balanced approach to conditioning training where aerobic/anaerobic ratios are close to equal.

Phase 3 athletes and those who guide them should take a close look at Table 5-3 in order to determine how to best approach their sport from a conditioning standpoint. If a youngster's priority sport is not included, use the percentages of a similar activity (i.e., softball/baseball) and estimate accordingly. Keep in mind that Phase 3 multi-sport athletes may have to shorten conditioning cycles because of lack of time and energy. Table 5-6 illustrates examples of proper conditioning protocols for Phase 3 athletes.

Types of Training	Duration/Distance	Speed/Intensity	Sets
Fartlek runs	30 to 45 minutes	Low/Medium/High	1
Interval sprints	200 to 500 meters	Medium/High	4
Slow, continuous aerobic activity	40 to 60 minutes	Low	1
Resisted sprints	40 to 60 meters	High	6

Table 5-6. Conditioning protocols for Phase 3 athletes

6

Youth Strength Training

Strength training, which for the purposes of this book will refer to moving resistance (body weight, barbells, dumbbells, machine plates, medicine balls, elastic bands, etc.) over a natural and safe range of motion, has undergone an extraordinary metamorphosis over the past half-century or so in the athletic community. Initially, it was an activity pursued only by the so-called "barbell competitors"—Olympic weight lifters, power lifters, and bodybuilders. Individual and team sport athletes, for the most part, avoided the weight room for fear of injury and performance deterioration.

Slowly but surely, however, the attitude toward strength training in the sports world began to shift. It started with athletes in pure power sports such as football, wrestling, and some field events (shot put, hammer throw, discus, etc.) as they cautiously dipped their toes into the strength training waters. What these competitors experienced was a shock to many. Strength training regularly actually seemed to improve their performance. They became bigger, stronger, faster, more explosive, and most important, better in their chosen sport.

With the genie out of the bottle, finesse athletes like baseball, basketball, and tennis players followed suit and began to hit the weights. Their experiences mirrored those of their powerful brethren: performance improved, injuries became less frequent, and overall physical prowess was enhanced.

It wasn't long after this that female athletes joined the strength-training fray. The majority of this group not only improved their ability to compete athletically, but found that their fears of becoming overly muscular (and thus losing their femininity) were misplaced. (Women, because of their biological make-up, do not have the capacity to build large amounts of muscle mass naturally). Strength training regularly has also proved to lower the incidence of series knee injuries among female athletes (see Chapter 3).

Which brings us to the last line of strength training resistance: young athletes. This sector of the sports community has been overrun with myths and untruths when it comes to lifting weights. Two of the most prominent (and erroneous) are that strength causes injury and stunts growth in youngsters. (Is it any wonder why youth coaches, fitness trainers, parents, and youngsters themselves have long had misgivings about strength training?)

Thankfully, as knowledge and common sense have prevailed, these concerns, along with many others, have proved unfounded. In fact, many of the myths relating to youth strength training have been shown not only to be untrue but the complete opposite of reality. For example, getting stronger through a properly designed strength-training program helps prevent injuries in young athletes, not cause them. And while strength training will not make athletes taller, per se, it does improve posture, which adds height when measured.

While strength training has demonstrated to be an appropriate and effective form of exercise for young athletes, it's important to re-emphasize to all involved that children are not merely smaller versions of mature adults. As such, precautions must be made and specialized strength training protocols implemented for safe and productive results. The following three chapters will address these protocols in detail.

What Strength Training Can Do for the Young Athlete

Strength training properly and regularly provides many positive byproducts for young athletes. It contributes to the prevention of injuries, as stronger muscles, joints, and bones are better able to withstand the rigors of participating in youth sports. Recent studies have shown that children who do some type of direct body-strengthening exercise are up to 50 percent less likely to incur injury on the playing field (court, ice, track, etc.) than those children who do not.

Strength training also improves sports performance in a number of ways. First and foremost, it increases the body's ability to generate force, which comes in handy when swinging a baseball or softball bat, executing a swimming stroke, or kicking a soccer ball. This enhanced force generation improves speed, quickness, and jumping ability as well, since a more powerful lower body allows for faster, more explosive sport-specific movements to be accomplished.

Increased strength and power in the core area (mid-section, lower back, and hips) developed through exercises like abdominal crunches, back raises, and deep squats will improve balance and agility, which are the key components in the ability to change direction at high speeds. Think of dodging a defender in lacrosse, avoiding a collision on the football field, or negotiating between two opponents in route to a lay-up in basketball. These activities, along with many others in a variety of sports, require the athlete to make split second decisions on which way to move. A strong center of gravity allows for this.

Strength training also has a positive effect on a child's stamina and endurance. Stronger muscles act more efficiently, allowing youngsters to continue demanding physical activities for longer periods of time without experiencing performance deterioration. Additionally, young athletes who participate in organized, year-round strength programs typically maintain high performance levels over numerous consecutive months and seasons while their less trained counterparts do not. This ability has become extremely important in recent years, as more and more young athletes are multi-sport participants.

Youngsters who strength train regularly enhance their capacity to absorb contact. Many sports (such as football, field hockey, and basketball, just to name a few) require the competitor to execute athletic skills while absorbing contact or collisions numerous times during a game. Increased overall body strength and stability will allow the young athlete to perform the requisite skills of their sport (i.e., catching a football across the middle, shooting a basketball in traffic, skiing down a mogul-filled mountain, etc.,) while under physical duress.

As youngsters enter into their early and mid-teen years, strength training will help to improve their body composition (ratio of muscle, bone, and fat in the body). A little-known fact outside of the fitness world is that building additional muscular body mass contributes to the burning of body fat. Simply put, the more muscle a young athlete has on his frame the more body fat he will burn during everyday activities. Imagine shredding unwanted fat while watching TV or sleeping—not a bad deal.

Pumping iron in a group setting also promotes camaraderie among young athletes. The weight room is a place where youngsters can workout in a congenial atmosphere away from the stress of competition and the critical eye of coaches. This type of interaction will lead to close, positive friendships that, in many cases, will last long after sports careers are concluded.

Finally, and perhaps the most important benefit of strength training, is that it engenders self-confidence. As young athletes become stronger, and eventually more muscular, they feel better about themselves and their bodies, which opens the gate to maximum athletic performance and achievement. Strength training will consistently yield plenty of other rewards, but the aforementioned should be enough to get youngsters into the weight room.

Youth Strength Training Basics

Before a strength-training program can be implemented for youngsters, all involved must first become familiar with the basics and principles of youth strength training. The following information will get young athletes started on the right track with their strength training workouts.

Strength Training Equipment

Youngsters will incorporate a variety of strength training equipment in their workout routines. The most popular and useful are discussed in the following section.

Barbells. Barbells are plate-loading bars that allow lifters to perform a variety of strength-training exercises such as bench presses, squats, and push presses. Weight plates ranging from 2.5 lbs. to 100 lbs. can be added or subtracted incrementally as needed. Olympic bars are the most widely used equipment of this type and can be seen racked on top of most conventional exercise benches in any gym or workout facility. They measure seven feet in length and weigh 45 pounds. Shorter, lighter versions are available for youngsters whose strength level does not yet warrant the use of a 45-pound Olympic bar. EZ curl barbells are also incorporated by many trainers for a variety of arm movements, as well as for the popular shoulder strengthening upright row exercise. These bars are indented for easy gripping and allow for a greater range of motion when executing some strength movements. All barbell exercises should be performed with collars fastened securely. Barbell training will begin for youngsters when they reach Phase 2.

Dumbbells. The best way to describe dumbbells is that they resemble miniature barbells and are designed to be handled in one hand either singularly (i.e., with dumbbell rows) or in unison (i.e., with dumbbell incline presses.) They range in weight from five to 150 pounds and are available in solid steel, non-adjustable plate, adjustable plate-loading, and rubberized varieties. Dumbbells are perhaps the most functional of all resistance-training equipment. They allow for a full range of motion (something that can't be said for barbells, exercise machines, or elastic bands), afford trainers an almost unlimited scope of strength-training exercises, and discourage compensation by the stronger limb, thus promoting balanced strength and muscular development. Dumbbells are also less cumbersome than most other strength training equipment and are therefore preferred for home use by many trainers. This equipment will be incorporated in all phases of a young athletes strength development program.

Weight machines. Strength training machines have become extremely popular throughout the sports conditioning world over the past two decades. Most elite athletes incorporate them at least partially in their strength-training routines. There are a large variety of strength-training machines available for use—including pulley, plate-loading, pin adjustable, and air resistance. Most styles offer many of the same basic strength-training exercises (lat pull-down, bench press, leg press, triceps press-down, arm curl, etc.) Regardless of strength machine type, the resistance runs along a predetermined track, enabling trainers to control the movement to a much greater degree than is possible with free weights. This feature may help beginning strength trainers to master proper exercise form. Many strength-training experts feel, however, that because the balancing aspect is eliminated, machine strength training is not nearly as effective for building overall body strength as is free weight training.

Unfortunately, some weight machines are too big for young athletes, especially those in Phase 1 of their athletic development. As such, machine strength training may not be an option for youngsters of small stature. In recent years, however, because of the popularity of youth strength training, equipment manufacturers have introduced a number of smaller strength training machines to accommodate smaller youngsters safely. These smaller versions are beginning to be more readily available in gyms, fitness facilities, and schools.

Medicine balls. Medicine balls are weighted spheres that come in a large variety of weights, sizes, and colors. They are incorporated in many conditioning disciplines including strength training. Rubber medicine balls are recommended for youngsters because they grip easily, bounce evenly when dropped, and are generally safer to use.

Elastic bands. Elastic bands, originally used exclusively for injury rehabilitation, are tailor made for young children's (Phase 1) strength-training programs. They are safe, easy on the joints (very important for the youngest of young athletes), and fun to train with. Bands have also proved to be productive in building strength in novice trainers.

The bands themselves vary in length and tension and are easily attached to any stationary object, including under the exerciser's feet. They can be used for virtually any strength-training exercise with the exception of explosive movements (hang clean, high pull, etc.) where barbells or dumbbells are required. While elastic bands are useful strength-training tools for beginners, as youngsters mature and become stronger, barbells, dumbbells, and selected exercise machines will be the strength-training equipment of choice. However, bands can and should be used periodically by older youngsters for variety or if an injury prohibits the use of other equipment.

Benches. Young strength trainers will incorporate a number of basic exercise benches in their workouts. They include non-adjustable, free-standing; non-adjustable, rack attached; adjustable, free-standing; adjustable, rack attached; and decline. While youngsters will train on all of these benches at different points in their athletic/workout careers, the adjustable, free-standing bench is by far the most useful. In fact, a comprehensive strength workout can be achieved with just an adjustable bench and a pair appropriately weighted dumbbells.

Power racks. Power racks are solid steel structures used to accommodate heavy barbells for exercises such as squats, upright rows, shrugs, hang cleans, push presses, and curls. They include two adjustable metal parallel bars that are designed to catch the weight if dropped, thus adding a degree of safety to the previously mentioned movements.

Swiss balls. Swiss balls (or stability balls, as they're frequently called) are inflatable, soft rubber balls that come in a variety of sizes to accommodate trainers of all heights. They are extremely effective for abdominal training, as the ball's giving surface forces the mid-section to stabilize on every repetition. Many trainers also use Swiss balls when executing wall slides, along with a variety of prone and seated upper-body dumbbell exercises (shoulder presses, lateral raises, bench presses, etc.). Keep in mind that because of the stability element inherent to Swiss ball training, the weight incorporated will be somewhat less than when exercising on a conventional bench. For those interested in further details concerning Swiss ball training, numerous books are available in the marketplace that deal exclusively with the subject.

Weightlifting belts. Some trainers use weightlifting belts when executing heavy standing lifts (push presses, squats, dead lifts, etc.). Most are made of nylon or leather, and have a width of approximately four to six inches in the front and eight to 12 inches in the back.

Weightlifting gloves. Weightlifting gloves, according to some, provide the lifter with a better grip on the bar. They also prevent calluses from developing on the hands. The gloves themselves are made of leather, and usually extend up to the knuckles of each finger and thumb.

Lifting straps. Straps are mostly used by bodybuilders to prevent grip fatigue during exercises such as chin-ups and upright rows. Since grip strength is of paramount importance in numerous sports (i.e., softball, wrestling, hockey, and golf), straps should not be incorporated into a young athlete's strength-training workout.

Safety

When it comes to youth strength training, the saying "safety first" has never been more appropriate. Without a safe and organized workout environment, consistent strength gains are impossible and training-related injuries extremely likely. As such, coaches, trainers, parents, or any other adult involved in overseeing youth strength workouts and programs must make safety the number one priority. A variety of safety tips are discussed in detail in the following sections.

Always warm up. In order to reduce the chances of suffering a strength training related injury, youngsters must be sufficiently warmed up prior to each and every weight workout. Refer to Chapter 2 for information on warming up.

Practice proper form. Incorporating proper lifting form on all exercises is essential to successful, injury-free strength training. As such, it is imperative that all young athletes master correct lifting technique prior to commencing with a strength program.

Use spotters. Without exception, an experienced spotter must be on hand for all heavy lifts performed by youngsters. Neglecting this advice can result in serious injury. In addition to ensuring safety, a knowledgeable spotter can correct errors in lifting form and help young athletes get the most out of a strength-training set by providing just enough help on that final, strength-promoting repetition.

Avoid heavy singles. Young lifters are notorious for showing off in the weight room (and elsewhere). This proclivity may seem harmless to some (simply a good-natured way to express themselves and compete with their peers), but in reality it can lead to serious injury, especially when maximum weight, single-repetition lifts are the proving ground. In fact, as much as half of strength-training-induced injuries would be prevented if heavy singles were avoided. The powers that be in the NFL and NBA seem to agree with this line of thinking. Both leagues have done away with the one-repetition maximum bench press test during their scouting combines, instead requiring athletes to lift a predetermined weight (175 pounds in basketball, 225 pounds in football) for as many repetitions as possible.

Abstain from horseplay. Fooling around during strength-training sessions is absolutely forbidden. It not only wastes precious gym time, but it can be downright dangerous for the young athlete and those around him. In short, youngsters should save the horseplay for the playground and keep it serious in the weight room.

Replace all equipment after use. Youngsters should get in the habit of replacing equipment after they're finished with it. A weight room or training facility strewn with objects (weight plates, machine pins, dumbbells, etc.) becomes a full blown injury trap.

Youth Strength Training Principles

Sets and repetitions. Sets and repetitions are the units of measure used in strength training. For example, shoulder pressing a pair of dumbbells 12 consecutive times with only a brief pause in-between lifts constitutes one set of 12 repetitions. The simple notation used to indicate such an effort is 1 x 12. The first number listed represents sets and the second figure represents repetitions.

Multi-joint exercises. Multi-joint exercises work more than one muscle group at a time. An example of a multi-joint lift is the squat, which exercises a variety of muscles, including the quadriceps, hips, lower back, and hamstrings. These movements will be the focal point of all phases of youth strength training.

Single-joint exercises. Sometimes referred to as auxiliary exercises, single-joint movements exercise one muscle group at a time. Two examples of single-joint exercises are barbell curls for the biceps and leg extensions for the quadriceps. These exercises will supplement multi-joint movements in a young athlete's strength program.

Combination exercises. Combination movements are complicated, multi-joint exercises that are designed to be performed in an explosive manner. Some examples of combination lifts include hang cleans, power cleans, and high pulls. With the exception of dead lifts, which can be performed at a controlled rate of speed, these exercises will only be incorporated by Phase 3 athletes who have developed a high level of strength, flexibility, and conditioning.

Train larger muscles first. It is important that young athletes train their muscles from largest to smallest during all strength workouts. Two basic reasons are behind this idea. First, the smaller muscle is already the weak link in the strength chain when executing any multi-joint lift. For example, in the squat, training the lower back prior to squatting would further weaken the smaller muscle (lower back), thus limiting the workload for the larger, stronger muscle groups (hips and quadriceps). Second, large body parts (upper back, chest, hips, etc.) require much more energy to train than do smaller muscle groups (calves, biceps, forearms, etc.). Therefore, it stands to reason that large muscle groups be exercised first in a strength workout when energy is at its highest.

Pyramid sets. For most effective results from strength training efforts, young athletes should incorporate pyramid sets into their workouts. Doing so entails gradually progressing from lighter weight sets to the heaviest set, then lowering the resistance on the final few sets. The notation might look something like this: 1 x 12, 1 x 10, 1 x 6, 1 x 8, 1 x 10.

Strength progression. Obviously, the major premise of a youth strength-training program is progression. To encourage this, it is best to perform the majority of sets (not including warm-up sets) near the point of muscular failure. For instance, if a program calls for a 10-repetition set, the youngster would chose a weight that allows him to complete 10 repetitions and no more. When more than 10 repetitions can be executed in good form, it is time to add weight. Usually a five-percent increase in weight is sufficient for multi-joint lifts.

Of course, finding the appropriate resistance level for each exercise in a young athlete's program will require a period of trial and error. Keep in mind that strength progression usually comes quite quickly for beginners. It is not atypical for a novice trainer to make substantial gains in strength in as little as three months. Sadly, as time moves forward and the body becomes accustomed to the rigors of strength training, increases become more difficult. Progression is still possible, however, albeit at a slower pace, and should always remain the priority.

Routine splitting. The split routine was first introduced in the bodybuilding community as a way for bodybuilders to exercise each body part with full energy at their disposal. It entails breaking the body's muscle groups into two or three separate sections and training each section with individual workouts. This technique will only apply to Phase 3 athletes, with the split consisting of one workout for the upper body and mid-section and another training session for the lower body and entire core region. While it is feasible to accomplish the two workouts on consecutive days, most young trainers respond best with a minimum of 48 hours rest between split sessions. Approaching the split routine in this manner will ensure optimum recovery.

Consistency. If youngsters hope to reach their strength potential, they must be consistent. In fact, consistency is so vital to the strength-building process that failure is not only possible without it, but assured. Young athletes should discipline themselves to get to the gym or workout facility regularly and then proceed to work hard when they get there. Even missing a few scheduled workouts can set youngsters back substantially. Lifting weights, perhaps more so than any other conditioning modality, is cumulative. The weight a young athlete lifts this week is directly correlated to the weight he lifted the previous week and so on down the line when it comes to developing strength, power, and muscle. No shortcuts and exceptions here.

Concentration. Concentration is an often-overlooked aspect of youth strength training. It is, however, of paramount importance. Youngsters of all ages must aspire to bring full concentration to every exercise, set, and repetition during their strength workouts. Maintaining full concentration, of course, is much easier said than done, given that the young mind can (and usually does) wander off in a million different directions. Unlike participating in a sporting event or team practice, where concentration comes about naturally due to outside stimuli, training with weights is a personal undertaking that requires constant, mindful attention. As such, all adult supervisors involved in youth strength-training programs should aspire to keep their charges focused on the task at hand in the weight room.

Breathing. Typically, young lifters will find it easier to inhale during the lowering phase of an exercise and breathe out during the lifting or work phase of the movement. Many athletes and trainers have found that, when working out with weights, their breathing tends to regulate naturally without much conscious thought. Obviously, youngsters should never hold their breath when strength training.

Rest between sets. How much a young athlete rests between strength-training sets depends largely on how heavy he is lifting. Since Phase 1 and Phase 2 youngsters will be training with light to medium loads their rest intervals will be fairly consistent, one-and-a-half to two minutes on average. Phase 3 trainers, on the other hand, will often engage in heavy training sessions, so up to 3 minutes recovery may be required under certain circumstances.

Lifting speed. When it comes to the speed of individual repetitions, many contrasting views exist. Some experts feel that lifting in a rapid fashion is more conducive to the needs of an athlete. Others believe that slower lifting allows a larger number of muscle fibers to come into play, thus ultimately developing more strength. Somewhere in the middle of these two camps is recommended for most youngsters. Unless a trainer is executing an explosive-type lift (hang clean, high pull, etc.) where high repetition speed is required or a specialized training technique like forced or negative repetitions where slow speed repetitions are employed, it is suggested that young athletes lift in a powerful, yet controlled, manner without sacrificing proper form.

Training the core. The power for all explosive athletic movements either emanates from or is transferred through the core of the body (mid-section, hips, and lower back). Because of this, it is the most important part of the physique when it comes to sports performance. A strong core also contributes to the prevention of a variety of injuries. Not surprisingly, core training will be a focal point of a young athlete's strength program.

Muscle balance. While some areas of the body are more essential to sports performance than others (i.e., the core region), it is nevertheless of paramount importance that balanced muscular development is achieved by all young athletes. When antagonist muscle groups, such as hamstrings and quadriceps, are out of balance strength wise, coordination and performance suffer and the risk of injury increases. This result is especially true in young female athletes, many of whom are prone to serious knee injuries because of an imbalance in strength between quadriceps (stronger) and hamstrings (weaker).

Free weights versus machines. The argument as to whether free weights or weight machines are superior for strength development has been debated for decades among bodybuilders, equipment manufactures, and authors of weight-training books. The fact is that a place exists for both in a young athlete's strength-training program. Free-weight exercises should, however, be the focal point in any competitive athlete's strength routine.

The most compelling reason why young athletes should build their strength programs around free weights, as opposed to machines, relates to the stabilizing muscles and joints (muscles and joints not directly involved in a particular the exercise). While not the prime movers, stabilizers help to balance and control the weight during an exercise. As such, working out with free weights stimulate these muscles and joints to a much greater degree than do machines, which, as mentioned previously, provide a predetermined path of movement. For instance, when comparing the back squat to the leg press, it is easy to see why the squat is the superior exercise. While both movements develop the quadriceps, hamstrings, and gluteal muscles, the squat indirectly strengthens the lower back, mid-section, shoulders, calves, ankles, wrists, and forearms. No machine ever invented has been able to duplicate this type of total body stimulation.

Additional reasons why free-weight training should be the strength workout modality of choice for aspiring athletes includes increased range of motion, variety of exercise choices, no size constraints, and the satisfaction and confidence component. (Lifting a loaded barbell off a rack and successfully imposing one's will against the resistance simply cannot be replicated by strapping oneself into a machine and moving a bar back and forth along a predetermined track.)

Of course, machines will not be neglected altogether in a young athlete's strength program. Many varieties such as the leg extension, leg curl, lat pull-down, leg press, pulley row, and triceps press-down are fundamental to any progressive resistance routine. Machines can be particularly effective for injury rehabilitation, as the movements are generally more controlled and less taxing on the joints. Also, beginners may find machine training helpful in learning proper exercise form. Finally, because changing poundage only requires moving a pin up or down a weight stack, as opposed to hauling big, cumbersome plates on and off a bar, machine workouts can be performed in less time than can free-weight sessions.

Where to strength train? Young athletes have numerous options when deciding where to take their strength workouts. Advantages and disadvantages apply to each. Various types of training facilities are reviewed in the following sections.

• Commercial health clubs. These clubs, or spas as they are sometimes called, cater to working men and women interested in becoming reasonably fit. They usually offer a wide variety of organized fitness classes (stretching, aerobics, spinning, yoga, body conditioning, etc.), and most provide whirlpools, saunas, massage treatment areas, and state-of-the-art shower facilities. The strength-training equipment also tends to be diverse and well maintained, although many commercial clubs emphasize glitzy machines over free weights.

The two main problems with commercial clubs is the relatively social atmosphere (not overly conducive to serious young athletes), and the large crowds, especially during post-work hours (5:30 pm to 8:30 pm). Anyone who has worked out in an crowed gym knows that getting your workout in as planned is extremely difficult, if not impossible. Be aware that many of these fancy health clubs are also very expensive, charging not only substantial monthly or yearly membership dues, but hefty initiation fees as well.

• Bodybuilding and power-lifting gyms. Bodybuilding and power-lifting gyms were the precursors to the health clubs mentioned in the previous section. Nothing fancy about these facilities—most are dimly lit, somewhat dingy looking places, with hundreds of pounds of free weights scattered about, and groups of very large, muscular men lifting copious amounts of iron.

While somewhat intimidating at first, hardcore weightlifting gyms can be fantastic places for young athletes to garner productive, strength-building workouts. The atmosphere of clanging weights and dedicated trainers can help motivate youngsters to outstanding efforts. An additional advantage of working out at one of these locations is the access to many experienced lifters, most of whom, despite their somewhat threatening appearance, are usually more than happy to impart their knowledge of weightlifting to novice and/or young trainers.

As with commercial clubs, bodybuilding and power-lifting facilities can get quite crowded at certain times of the day. This drawback is exacerbated by the relatively small size of these gyms (many are privately owned). Most have shower facilities, but don't expect fancy steam rooms or saunas. On balance, however, hardcore gyms are suggested over the health club variety for serious young athletes looking to reach ultimate levels of strength and power.

• Team-training centers. Young athletes who are fortunate enough to have access to a team-training center should take full advantage. Not only are these facilities usually well-equipped, but they provide youngsters the rare opportunity to interact with peers in a common purpose environment of becoming stronger, more powerful athletes. Additionally, most team-training centers employ at least one sports strength-training specialist to guide and supervise workouts, answer strength-training-related questions, and devise year-round strength programs for youngsters.

Unfortunately, many team-training centers are available only at certain times of year, perhaps just during the school term. Also, even if the facility is available, your teammates may not be due other commitments. Notwithstanding the problems with accessibility and logistics, a team-training center is (according to most sports strength-and-conditioning experts) the best location for youngsters to perform their strength training sessions.

• Home training. Strength training at home can give youngsters a tremendous amount of scheduling flexibility. If the preference is to workout at noon or midnight, the gym is always open (although at midnight, other members of the household may not agree that the gym should be open). Home training also provides novice trainers (who may be somewhat intimidated by a gym setting) a comfortable, self-contained atmosphere in which to work out and learn the basics of strength training. Finally, home-training sessions can usually be performed quickly with no waiting in line for equipment or long walks from one area of the gym to the other as would be the case at a commercial facility.

Although home strength training has many advantages (such as the ones detailed in the previous paragraph), there are some drawbacks. First, home gyms are usually small and unable to accommodate the variety of equipment that public facilities can. This limitation often leads to boredom, which can hinder strength development. Second, many young trainers find it hard to motivate themselves without the collective energy of a gym atmosphere; clanging weights and supportive voices keep these youngsters engaged and on track during workouts. Third, unless a training partner is on hand for all home workouts, the benefit of a spotter will not be present, a factor that can be strength restricting and dangerous.

Whether the home gym is the prime location for a young athlete's strength workouts or not, it is still strongly suggested that some basic strength training equipment be available at home. An adjustable bench, barbell and weight set, a pair of adjustable dumbbells, a chinning bar, and a few appropriately weighted medicine balls would be ideal. Having this equipment will come in handy regardless of where a youngster decides to take the majority of his strength workouts.

Record keeping. It is extremely important that young athletes maintain regular and accurate records concerning their strength training. Strength training program coordinators should encourage youngsters to keep their own records. Doing so will not only promote strength gains, but engender personal responsibility as well. Recommended entries in a training log include date of workouts, exercises, weight used, sets per exercise, repetitions per set, total sets per workout, rest between sets, and workout duration.

Variety. When it comes to strength training, exercise variety is a must. Mixing up a workout routine is essential to consistent progress. A number of reasons can be listed to support this factor.

First, changing a workout routine periodically keeps muscles off balance, forcing them to adjust to the new demands placed upon them, thus producing gains in strength, power, and (for Phase 3 athletes) muscle size. Young bodies adapt fairly quickly to exercise. As such, they must be constantly challenged with new stimuli in order to improve.

Second, incorporating different exercises, set sequences, repetition schemes, and training intensities enable workouts to be more interesting and creative. The tediousness of performing the same workout week after week and month after month can take its toll on the attitude of even the most dedicated young athlete.

Finally, being flexible with a strength-training program will help youngsters avoid overuse injuries. Working muscles and joints from the same angle with the same movements for an extended number of workouts will eventually lead to injury.

Limitations. No matter how great a young athlete's potential, at some point he will hit his strength, power, and muscular size limit. It may seem odd to bring up limitations in a book dedicated to the improvement of young athletes, but realizing individual limits is an important factor in getting the most out of a strength program. Having unrealistic expectations can be almost as dangerous to progress as setting lackluster goals. Youngsters must understand that genetics, like it or not, play a major role in muscle and strength development.

When not to strength train? Other than the obvious times (when injured, sick, overtrained, or on a planned training break), young athletes should abstain from strength training the day of and the day before an important sporting event in which they are participating. Strength training too close to competition can leave muscles sore and energy depleted—not exactly what performance-conscious young athletes are looking for. The only exception here is strength training immediately following competition, which can help the body cool down and is a great way to keep current with individual strength programs.

7

Strength Training Exercises

Body Weight and Core Exercises

Body Weight Squat

Muscles trained: Hips, quadriceps, buttocks, hamstrings, and lower back

Exercise type: Multi-joint

Movement execution: Standing with your feet approximately shoulder-width apart and pointed slightly outward, bend at the knees as if attempting to sit in a chair and lower yourself down until your upper legs are just below parallel to the floor. Keeping your head up and your back straight, drive yourself back up to the standing position. Hands can be positioned either at your sides or directly out in front of you.

Training tips and variations: When performing squats, it is important that your knees remain behind your toes throughout the movement. To increase difficulty, you can execute this exercise while wearing a weighted vest or holding a medicine ball at arm's length in front of you.

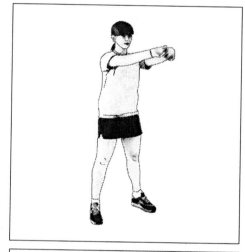

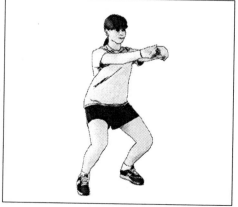

Push-Up

Muscles trained: Middle chest, anterior deltoids, and triceps

Exercise type: Multi-joint

Movement execution: Assume a conventional push-up position, which entails facing the floor with your head level, your hands planted firmly on the ground at approximately shoulder width and chest level, your legs fully extended, and your feet close together. Begin by rising up to the arms-extended position (starting position) and proceed by lowering yourself down until your chest is within a few inches of the floor. From the low position, powerfully push up by extending your arms to just short of the locked out position.

Training tips and variations: Push-ups can be made more difficult by raising your feet on a step or bench, closing your grip, wearing resistance equipment such as a weighted vest, or incorporating specially-designed push-up bars, which allow for increased range of motion. Advanced Phase 3 trainers can even try performing push-ups while grabbing hold of a medicine ball or some other unstable object. To lessen the intensity of the exercise, balance your lower body on your knees instead of your toes.

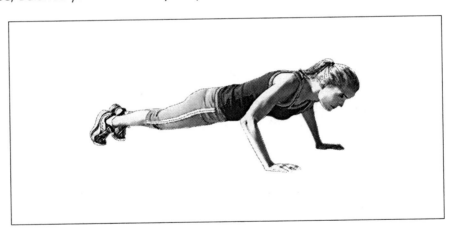

Body Weight Lateral Step-Up

Muscles trained: Hips, quadriceps, buttocks, hamstrings, and calves

Exercise type: Multi-joint

Movement execution: With your arms at your sides and your head up, step laterally up on to a box, bench, or step (the height of the box/bench/step will vary depending on the stature, strength, and athletic ability of the youngster involved) as if you were climbing stairs. Your arms will swing as if running in place during execution. Pause at the top with both legs straight and carefully step back down to the floor and repeat.

Training tips and variations: Phase 3 athletes can perform this exercise in an explosive manner.

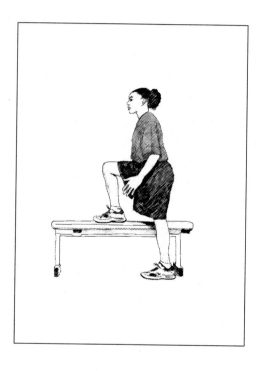
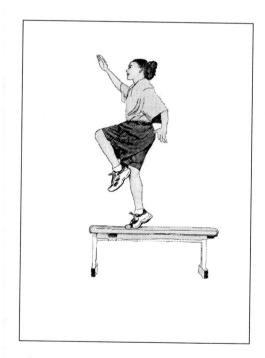

Inverted Chin-Up

Muscles trained: Latisimus dorsi, biceps, posterior deltoids, and forearms

Exercise type: Multi-joint

Movement execution: Place your heels on a raised surface such as an exercise bench or stability ball and hang at arms length with an overhand, shoulder width grip from a racked bar. Proceed to pull yourself up until the bar is directly under your chin. Lower under control to the starting position and repeat.

Training tips and variations: This exercise can be performed with an underhand grip for variety. A smith machine can be used in lieu of a conventional bar and bench.

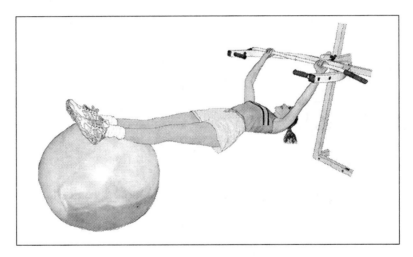

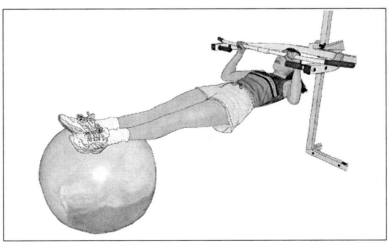

Dip

Muscles trained: Lower chest, anterior deltoids, and triceps

Exercise type: Multi-joint

Movement execution: Start by balancing at arm's length above a dipping bar or parallel bars. Lower yourself under control until your shoulders are slightly above the bars. Then push upward forcefully to the arms extended position.

Training tips and variations: To make dips more difficult, you can add resistance by wearing a weighted vest or placing a dumbbell between crossed ankles during execution. To lessen intensity, dips can be performed on a gravitron machine, where a percentage of your body weight can be used. Youngsters with a history of shoulder problems should abstain from dips.

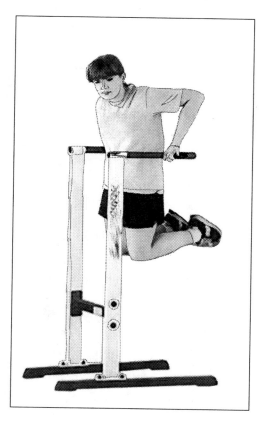 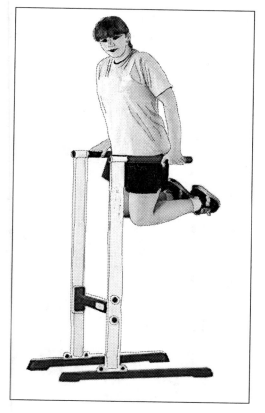

Chin-Up

Muscles trained: Upper latisimus dorsi, posterior deltoids, biceps, forearms

Exercise type: Multi-joint

Movement execution: Grab hold of a chinning bar with an overhand grip and hang down at arm's length. Your hands should be spaced several inches wider than shoulder width. Pull yourself up so that the bar touches your upper chest just below your chin. Proceed to lower yourself down under control to the arm's extended position.

Training tips and variations: When performing chin-ups, arching your back slightly during the concentric (pulling up) portion of the movement is suggested. This action will ensure that the upper back muscles are fully engaged. The chin-up exercise has many variations, including bringing the bar to the back of your neck, using an underhand grip, or incorporating a double-handled bar. Younger children may want to execute this movement on a gravitron, where a percentage of your body weight can be used, until their strength levels increase.

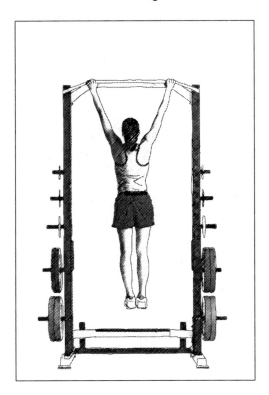 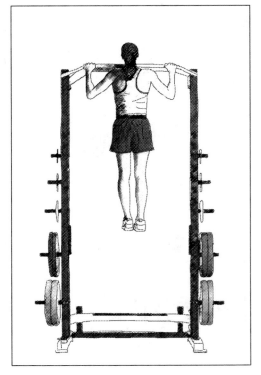

Bench Dip

Muscles trained: Triceps, entire shoulder girdle, lower chest

Exercise type: Multi-joint

Movement execution: Sit in the middle of an exercise bench with your hands at your sides and your legs extended in front of you. While balancing on your heels, proceed to lift yourself off the bench and then, by bending at the elbows, lower your body down as far as possible. Once in the low position, pause briefly and then powerfully push yourself up until your arms are fully extended.

Training tips and variations: Too add intensity to bench dips, place a light medicine ball or barbell plate on your lap during execution.

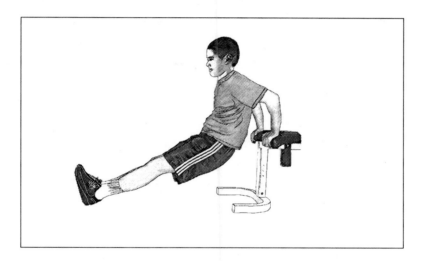

Wall Slide

Muscles trained: Quadriceps, hips, buttocks, and hamstrings

Exercise type: Multi-joint

Movement execution: Position your straight back against a wall with your knees bent at approximately 120 degrees and your feet planted firmly on the floor, positioned slightly wider than shoulder width. With your back maintaining contact with the wall, slide slowly down until your upper legs are just below parallel to the floor. Pause for a five count at the bottom and then proceed to push yourself back up to the starting position.

Training tips and variations: Wall slides can be executed with a Swiss ball positioned between the wall and the youngster's back (see illustration). To increase intensity of this exercise, hold an appropriately-weighted medicine ball or dumbbell at arms length directly out in front of you during execution.

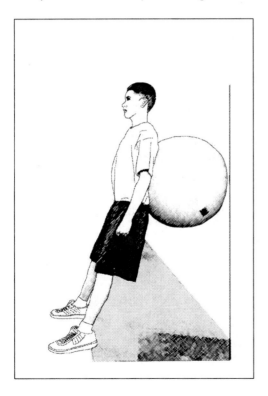 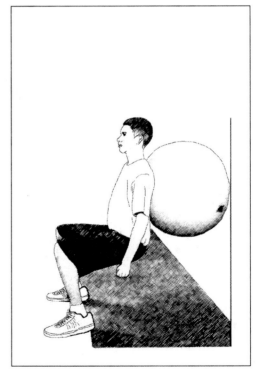

Bench Crunch

Muscles trained: Upper abdominal region

Exercise type: Single-joint

Movement execution: Lying on your back with your hands clasped behind your head, place your feet and lower legs over a flat exercise bench. Proceed to sit up, raising your head toward your knees. Pause momentarily at the top of the movement and then lower your body under control back down to the floor.

Training tips and variations: This exercise can be executed without a bench by placing feet flat on the floor with your legs bent at the knees. Numerous machines also simulate the crunching motion; however most are not nearly as effective as the floor version. For added intensity, place a barbell plate or medicine ball behind your head during execution.

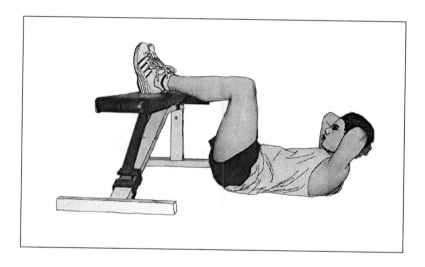

Straight-Legged Toe Touch

Muscles trained: Lower abdominal region

Exercise type: Single-joint

Movement execution: Lying on your back with your arms extended upward, hold your legs straight in the air as high as possible. From there, reach up and touch your toes, as you simultaneously contract your lower abdominal muscles.

Training tips and variations: For best results, straight-legged toe touches should be performed in a quick, explosive manner.

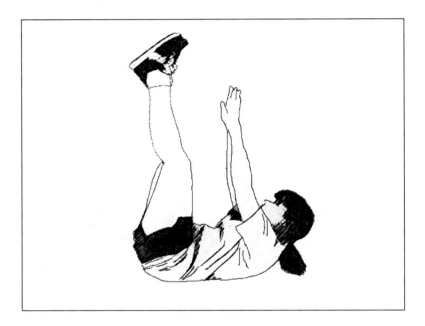

Navy Seal Kicks

Muscles trained: Lower abdominal region

Exercise type: Single-joint

Movement execution: Lie flat on your back with your arms behind your head. Begin by raising your hips slightly and then proceed to kick your legs repetitively straight up and down without your feet touching the floor for the required time or number of repetitions.

Training tips and variations: For increased support when performing navy seal kicks, grab on to a stationary object positioned at arms length above your head. To increase intensity, a pair of light ankle weight can be worn during execution.

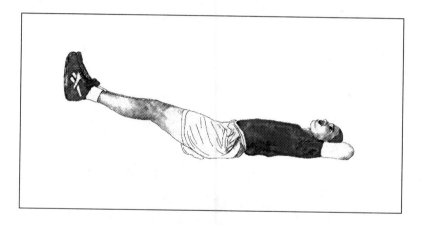

Ball Twist

Muscles trained: Entire abdominal region and obliques

Exercise type: Single-joint

Movement execution: Lie on your back with your knees slightly bent and raise your feet off the floor approximately six inches. Grab either a basketball, volleyball, or a soccer ball and hold it at your mid-section a few inches above your body. Then, while keeping your knees bent and your legs off the floor, raise your torso up until you're balancing on your tailbone. Proceed to swing from your mid-section and touch the ball to the floor. Continue back and forth for the required number of repetitions.

Training tips and variations: Stronger Phase 3 youngsters can substitute a medicine ball for this exercise. To lessen the intensity of ball twists, plant your feet firmly on the ground during execution.

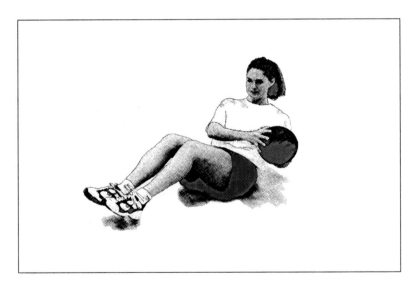

Bicycle Sit-Up

Muscles trained: Entire abdominal region and obliques

Exercise type: Single-joint

Movement execution: Lying on your back with your hands lightly touching the back of your head and your legs two to three feet off of the ground, proceed to sit-up, while simultaneously bringing your right elbow to your left knee. Return to the starting position and repeat by bringing your left elbow to your right knee. Continue to alternate in this manner for the required number of repetitions.

Training tips and variations: Some advanced Phase 3 athletes may want to incorporate a medicine ball for this exercise by moving it from knee to knee during execution.

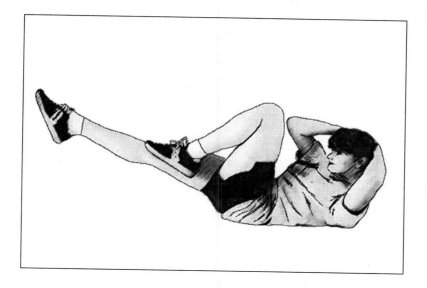

Hip-Up

Muscles trained: Lower abdominal region

Exercise type: Single-joint

Movement execution: Begin by lying on your back on a flat exercise bench and bring your knees to your chest. Next, take hold of the bench with both hands positioned behind your head. Proceed to drive your hips and legs up in the air as high as you can. Pause briefly at the top and then return to the starting position.

Training tips and variations: If a bench is not available, hip-ups can be performed on the floor while grabbing a stationary object with both hands behind your head. Some advanced youngsters may want to add resistance to this exercise by wearing a pair of light ankle weights during execution.

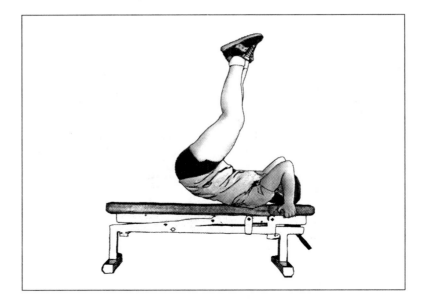

Hanging Leg Raise

Muscles trained: Lower abdominal region

Exercise type: Single-joint

Movement execution: Start by hanging at arm's length from a chinning bar with an overhand, shoulder-width grip. Proceed to lift your legs straight out in front of you, while maintaining stationary hips. Hold for a count at the top and then return your legs to the starting position.

Training tips and variations: This movement can also be performed on a vertical bench, where you support yourself by the elbows, thus taking the grip element out of the exercise. To lessen intensity, youngsters can bend their knees during the up phase of the movement.

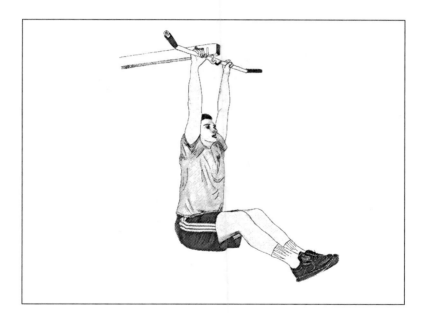

Floor Back Raise

Muscles trained: Entire lower back region

Exercise type: Single-joint

Movement execution: Lying face down on the floor, slowly raise your legs and trunk in unison as high as possible. Hold for a two count at the contracted position and then slowly lower yourself back to down to the floor.

Training tips and variations: Floor back raises can be executed by raising one leg and one arm at a time (left leg, right arm; right leg, left arm) for variety.

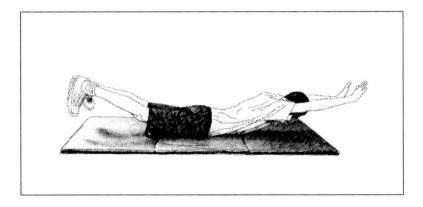

Prone Hyper-Extension

Muscles trained: Entire lower back region and upper hamstrings

Exercise type: Multi-joint

Movement execution: Position yourself so that you are face down across a hyper-extension bench, with your feet securely underneath the footpads. With your arms folded across your chest, bend straight down from the waist over the pad. Pause briefly in the low position, and then come back up under control until your torso is just above parallel to the floor.

Training tips and variations: Some trainers prefer to position their hands behind their necks as opposed to across their chests when performing prone hyper-extensions. For older, stronger young athletes, resistance can be added by holding a barbell plate, dumbbell, or medicine ball across the chest.

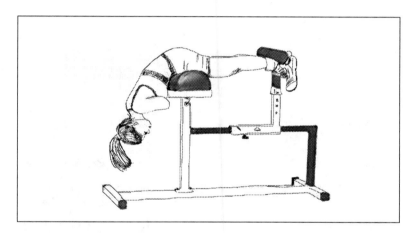

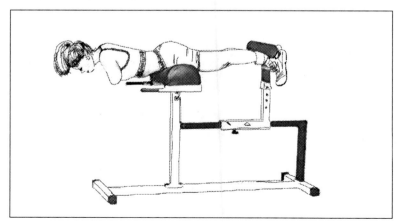

Good Morning

Muscles trained: Entire lower back region and hamstrings

Exercise type: Multi-joint

Movement execution: Standing with your feet close together, hold an appropriately-weighted barbell behind your neck. Keeping your legs and back straight, bend at the waist until your upper body is parallel to the floor. Pause briefly, and then rise up under control back to the standing position.

Training tips and variations: Phase 1 youngsters will perform good mornings with either a broomstick or light medicine ball in lieu of a barbell.

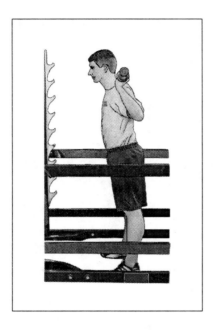 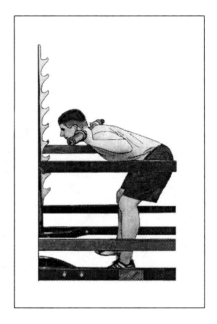

Reverse Back Raise

Muscles trained: Entire lower back region

Exercise type: Single-joint

Movement execution: Lean over a hyper-extension bench so that the pad supports your mid-section and pelvis. (You'll be facing the opposite direction as you would during prone hyper-extensions.) Grab the rollers with both hands and let your legs hang down naturally. Proceed to lift your legs and pelvis in a controlled motion until they are slightly higher than your lower back. Hold for a count and then return to the starting position.

Training tips and variations: Some advanced Phase 3 athletes can add resistance to reverse back raises by wearing ankle weights or holding a light dumbbell between their ankles.

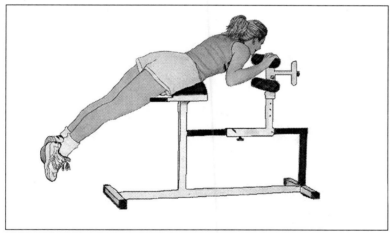

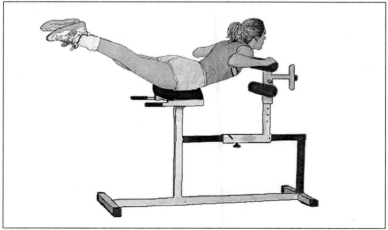

Upper Body Exercises

Bench Press

Muscles trained: Middle chest, anterior deltoids, and triceps

Exercise type: Multi-joint

Movement execution: Lying on your back on a flat exercise bench with your hands slightly wider than shoulder width, lift a loaded barbell off a rack and hold it with your arms extended above you. With your feet planted firmly on the ground and your buttocks tight to the bench, lower the weight under control to mid-chest level. Pause briefly and proceed to press the bar back up to the locked out position.

Training tips and variations: It is important that you keep your back as flat as possible to the bench when bench pressing (no arching). Arching increases the risk of injury substantially. This exercise can be performed with dumbbells and on a variety of machines.

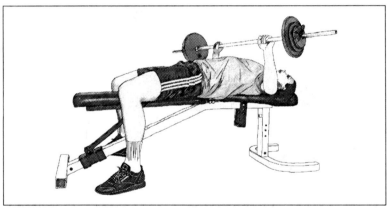

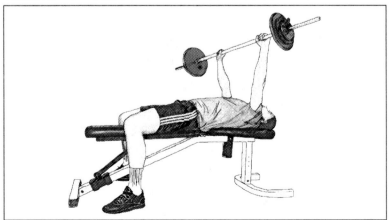

Incline Dumbbell Press

Muscles trained: Upper chest, anterior deltoids, and triceps

Exercise type: Multi-joint

Movement execution: Lying on a free-standing incline bench (at approximately a 45-degree incline), grab hold of two appropriately-weighted dumbbells and position them at shoulder height with elbows out at your sides and palms facing forward. Proceed to press the dumbbells up in unison to the arms locked position.

Training tips and variations: It is important when performing incline presses to avoid the tendency to press the weights out instead of up. The resistance should be pressed straight up on each and every repetition. The incline press can be performed with a barbell and on a variety of machines.

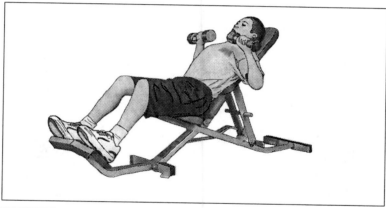

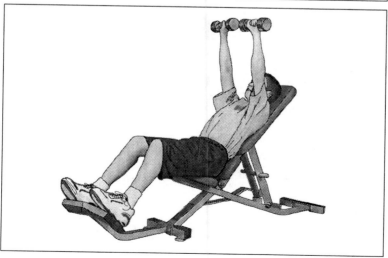

Cable Crossover

Muscles trained: Middle chest

Exercise type: Single-joint

Movement execution: Stand with your knees flexed, and while leaning slightly forward at the waist, grab hold of the handles of an overhead cable pulley machine. Proceed to bring your hands together in a hugging motion until they touch. Pause briefly, and slowly return the handles to the starting position.

Training tips and variations: Cable crossovers can be a somewhat awkward exercise. As such, younger athletes (Phase 1 and early Phase 2) should use very little weight when executing this movement.

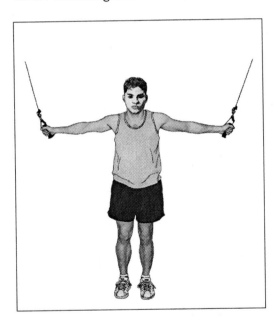 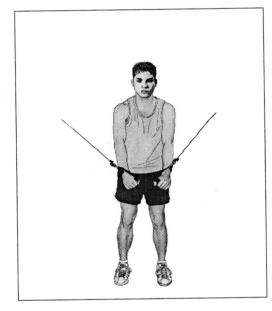

Dumbbell Shoulder Press

Muscles trained: Anterior deltoids, medial deltoids, and triceps

Exercise type: Multi-joint

Movement execution: Seated on a flat exercise bench, grab hold of an appropriately-weighted dumbbell in each hand and position them at shoulder height with elbows out at your sides and palms facing forward. Proceed to lift the dumbbells straight up to the arm's extended position, hold for a count, and then lower the resistance back to the starting position.

Training tips and variations: This exercise can be performed with a barbell or on a variety of machines. If shoulder or neck problems exist, however, barbell shoulder presses should be avoided.

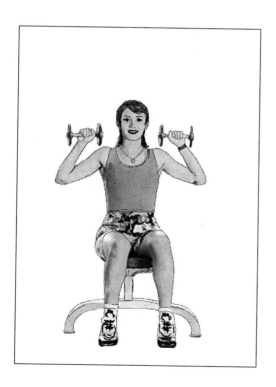 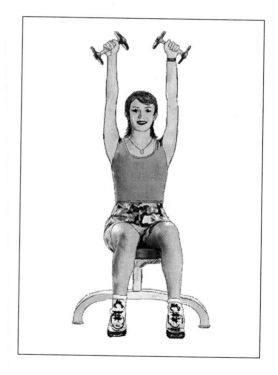

Dumbbell Upright Row

Muscles trained: Trapezius, medial deltoids, posterior deltoids, biceps, and forearms

Exercise type: Multi-joint

Movement execution: In a standing position, grasp two appropriately-weighted dumbbells with an overhand grip. Starting with your arms hanging down, lift the resistance straight up, keeping the dumbbells as close to your body as possible, to a point just below your chin. Pause briefly in the contracted position and then lower the weights slowly back down to the starting position.

Training tips and variations: Upright rows can be performed with a barbell, a floor pulley, or on a Smith machine for variety.

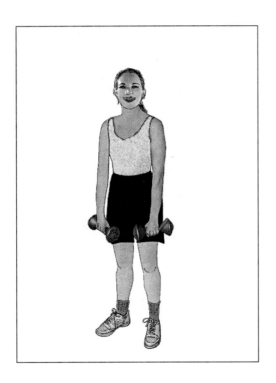 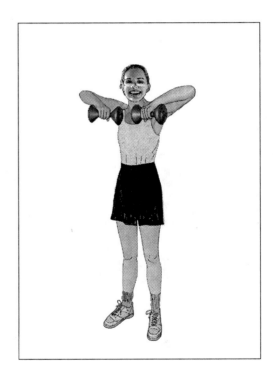

Lateral Raise

Muscles trained: Medial deltoids

Exercise type: Single-joint

Movement execution: Standing with your knees slightly flexed, take hold of two moderately-weighted dumbbells and position them at your sides. Keeping your elbows slightly bent, proceed to raise the weights in unison away from your sides, until your arms are just above parallel to the ground. Lower the dumbbells slowly back to the starting position.

Training tips and variations: Lateral raises can also be executed seated. A number of machines can be used for this exercise as well.

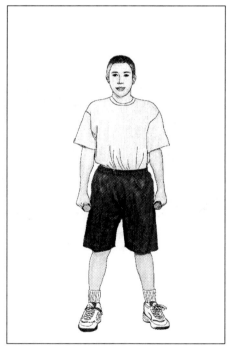 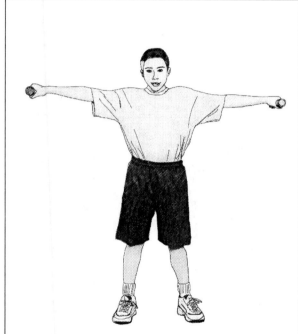

Bent Lateral Raise

Muscles trained: Posterior deltoids

Exercise type: Single-joint

Movement execution: Seated near the end of a flat exercise bench, lean over at the waist and grab two light dumbbells from the floor. Keeping your body balanced and your head down, lift the weights out to either side, turning your wrists so that your thumbs are pointed downward, until both dumbbells are just above head height. Return the resistance under control to the starting position.

Training tips and variations: For best results, bent lateral raises should be performed with relatively light weights. This exercise can be executed standing while bending at the waist, prone over a 45-degree incline bench, or on a variety of machines.

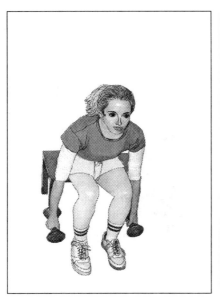 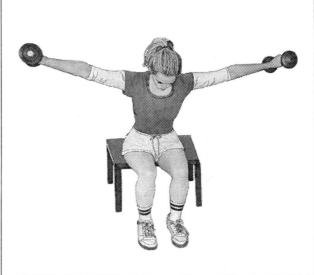

Internal Rotation

Muscles trained: Rotator cuff

Exercise type: Single-joint

Movement execution: Lie on your back on a flat exercise bench and take hold of a light dumbbell in one hand. Keeping your arm bent at a 90-degree angle, rotate it inward to your lower chest. Return to the low position and repeat.

Training tips and variations: This exercise can also be performed with an elastic band from a standing position.

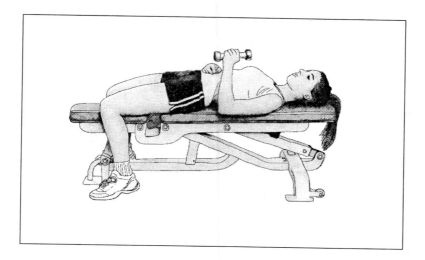

External Rotation

Muscles trained: Rotator cuff

Exercise type: Single-joint

Movement execution: Lie on your side on a flat exercise bench and take hold of a light dumbbell with your upper hand. Keeping your arm bent at a 90-degree angle and your elbow tucked to your upper hip, rotate it upward. Return to the starting position and repeat.

Training tips and variations: This exercise can also be performed with an elastic band from a standing position.

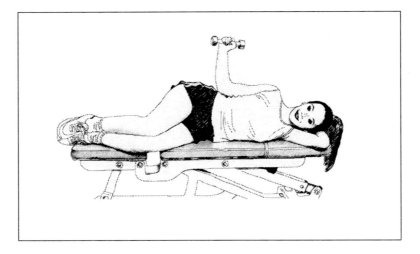

Pull-Down

Muscles trained: Upper latisimus dorsi, posterior deltoids, biceps, and forearms

Exercise type: Multi-joint

Movement execution: Incorporating a lat machine, grab the bar with a fairly wide, overhand grip. Then, arching your back slightly, pull the bar down until it touches the top of your chest just below your neck. Pause briefly and proceed to extend your arms back to the starting position.

Training tips and variations: Similar to chin-ups, it is possible to incorporate a variety of hand placements when performing pull-downs. Unlike chin-ups, you can exercise with less than your body weight.

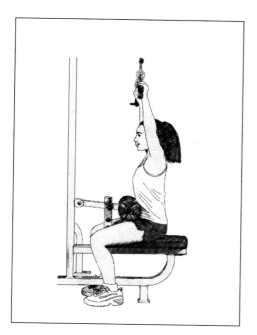 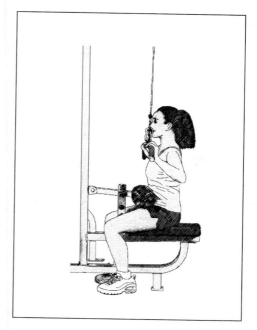

Dumbbell Row

Muscles trained: Middle and lower latisimus dorsi, posterior deltoids, biceps, and forearms

Exercise type: Multi-joint

Movement execution: Place one hand and one knee on a flat exercise bench. Grab hold of a sufficiently heavy dumbbell from the floor and, keeping your back flat and your grounded foot firmly based, lift the weight up to your side. Pause briefly at the top of the movement and then lower the resistance under control back to the floor.

Training tips and variations: Because the lower back is supported during the execution of dumbbell rows, it is possible to incorporate very heavy weights in this exercise without fear of injury. This movement can also be performed on a variety of machines, however, the dumbbell version is far superior for strength development.

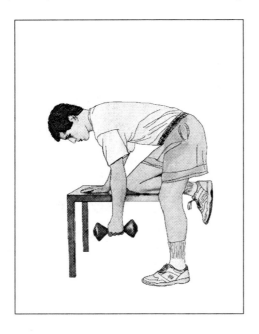 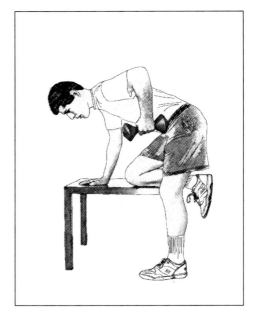

Seated-Cable Row

Muscles trained: Lower latisimus dorsi, posterior deltoids, biceps, and forearms

Exercise type: Multi-joint

Movement execution: Seated in a cable-row apparatus, grip the handle firmly with both hands and position your feet firmly on the raised platform in front of you. With your knees partially bent, proceed to lower the weight to the arms-extended position (i.e., starting position). Then, pull the resistance back toward your body, arching your back slightly, and touch the handle to your abdomen. Continue by slowly returning the weight to the starting position.

Training tips and variations: The negative (lowering) phase of seated-cable rows should be performed in a very controlled fashion. Doing so will allow you to fully stretch the back muscles, thus producing optimum strength building results. The lower back is not supported during this exercise. As such, youngsters with lower back problems should abstain from seated-cable rows.

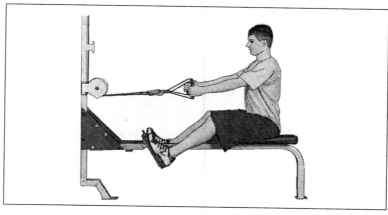

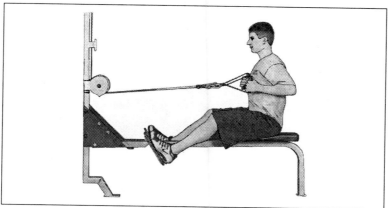

Triceps Press Down

Muscles trained: Triceps

Exercise type: Single-joint

Movement execution: Grasp a short bar from an overhead pulley with a close, overhand grip. With your elbows close to your torso and your knees slightly flexed, push the bar down, locking your elbows at the bottom. Release and bring the resistance down under control to mid-chest level and repeat.

Training tips and variations: Triceps press downs can be performed using a v-shaped bar, a specially-designed rope, or on a lat machine for variety. An underhand grip can be incorporated for added stretch.

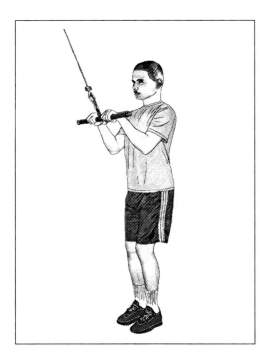 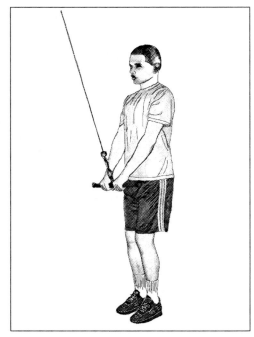

Lying Triceps Extension

Muscles trained: Triceps

Exercise type: Single-joint

Movement execution: Lying on a flat exercise bench with your head just off the edge, take hold of an appropriately-weighted barbell with a slightly closer than shoulder-width grip and place it just above your forehead. Keeping your elbows stationary, push the weight up by extending your arms to the locked out position. Then, carefully lower the bar back to the starting position.

Training tips and variations: Many trainers feel that using an E-Z curl bar when performing lying triceps extensions provides more control and a slightly increased range of motion. If an exercise bench is not available, it is possible to execute this exercise while lying flat on the floor.

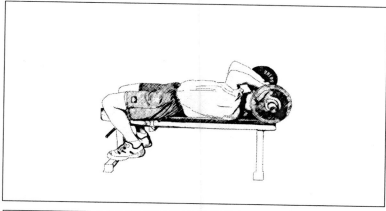

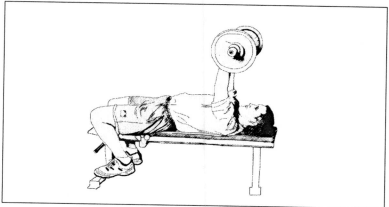

Seated Triceps Extension

Muscles trained: Triceps

Exercise type: Single-joint

Movement execution: Sit on the end of a flat exercise bench and grasp a barbell overhand with your hands six to eight inches apart. Bring the weight behind your head until your upper arms are approximately parallel to the floor (starting position). Then, extend your arms, pushing the bar overhead to the locked out position.

Training tips and variations: Phase 1 athletes will incorporate dumbbells for seated triceps extensions. This exercise can also be performed from a standing position.

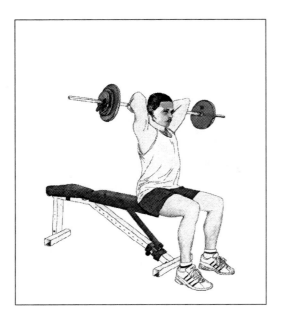 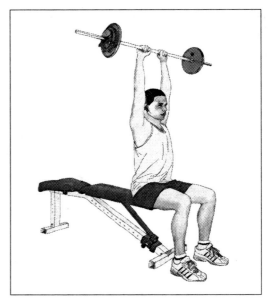

Dumbbell Kick-Back

Muscles trained: Triceps

Exercise type: Single-joint

Movement execution: Grab two light dumbbells and stand with your knees slightly flexed and your upper body leaning over until it is parallel to the ground. With your back remaining straight, extend your arms straight back, keeping your elbows stationary throughout.

Training tips and variations: Kick-backs can be performed with two ground based pulleys or elastic bands for variety.

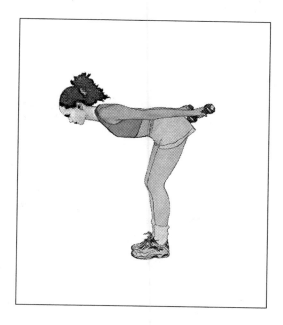

Standing Curl

Muscles trained: Biceps

Exercise type: Single-joint

Movement execution: Standing with your knees slightly flexed, grab hold of a barbell with an underhand, shoulder-width grip. Let the bar hang down with your arms straight and then, with your back straight and elbows close to your torso, curl the weight up smoothly to your upper chest. Pause at the top and proceed to lower the resistance back down to the starting position.

Training tips and variations: In order to squeeze out a few extra repetitions, a small amount of body swing is acceptable during standing curls. Phase 1 athletes will incorporate dumbbells for this exercise.

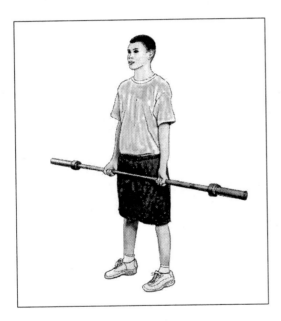 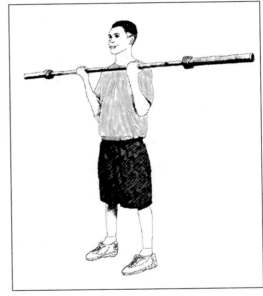

Incline Dumbbell Curl

Muscles trained: Upper biceps

Exercise type: Single-joint

Movement execution: Seated on an incline bench, hold an appropriately weighted dumbbell in each hand with your arms fully extended and your palms facing each other. With your elbows in, curl both dumbbells in unison, while slowly twisting your palms upward, to your front deltoids. Lower the weights under control back to the starting position.

Training tips and variations: It is important that you pause at the bottom of the movement to prevent momentum from becoming a factor in the next repetition. Dumbbells can lifted one at a time for variety.

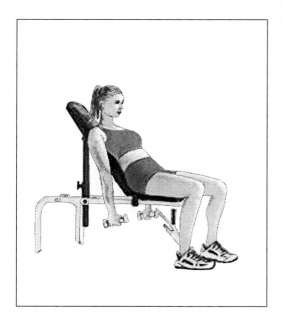 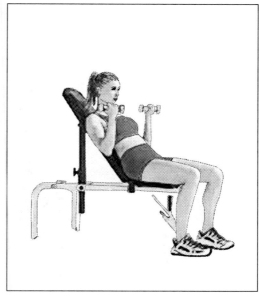

Preacher Curl

Muscles trained: Lower biceps

Exercise type: Single-joint

Movement execution: Seated on a preacher bench with your chest against the pad, grasp a barbell with an underhand grip from the rack. Your hands should be spaced approximately eight to 10 inches apart. Without rocking backward, curl the bar up to just under forehead height. Pause briefly and slowly return the resistance back to the arms extended position.

Training tips and variations: When performing preacher curls, many experienced weight lifters feel that squeezing the biceps muscles at the top of the movement adds to strength and muscular development. Phase 1 youngsters will incorporate dumbbells for this exercise. A variety of machines simulate the preacher curl; however, the free-weight version is far superior for strength development.

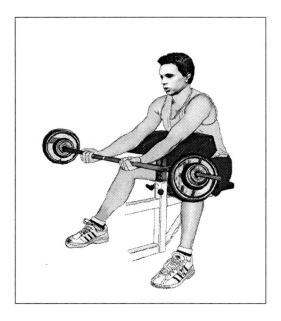 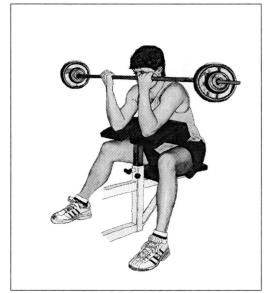

Hammer Curl

Muscles trained: Forearms and biceps

Exercise type: Single-joint

Movement execution: Seated at the end of a flat exercise bench, grasp a reasonably light dumbbell in each hand. With your arms fully extended at your sides and your palms facing each other, curl the weights straight up to your front deltoids, maintaining stationary wrists throughout. Pause at the top and then lower the weights under control back to the starting position.

Training tips and variations: Hammer curls can also be performed standing.

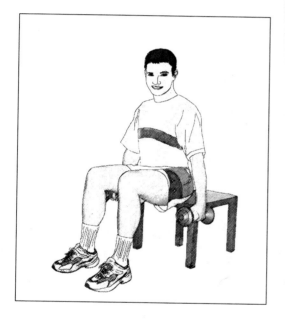 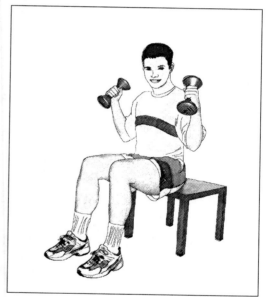

Wrist Roller

Muscles trained: Forearms

Exercise type: Single-joint

Movement execution: Stand with your arms extended directly in front of you holding the ends of a wrist roller with an overhand grip. With the weight hanging down and the line taut, proceed to roll the resistance up using the strength in your forearms and wrists. When the weight reaches the top, slowly unroll the line and repeat.

Training tips and variations: For variety, you can hold the wrist roller with an underhand grip.

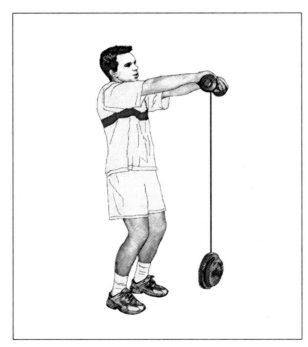

Lower Body and Combination Exercises

Squat

Muscle trained: Hips, quadriceps, buttocks, hamstrings, and lower back

Exercise type: Multi-joint

Movement execution: Standing with your feet approximately shoulder-width apart and pointed slightly outward, rest a loaded barbell across your shoulders behind your neck. With your hands balancing the bar, bend your knees as if attempting to sit in a chair and lower yourself until your upper legs are just below parallel to the floor. Keeping your head up and your back straight, drive yourself back up to the standing position.

Training tips and variations: When performing squats, it is important that your knees remain behind your toes throughout the movement. Not doing so leaves you vulnerable to knee stress. Also, newcomers to strength training should incorporate very light weight in the squat until they become comfortable with the exercise. Dumbbells resting on the front of the shoulders can be used in lieu of a barbell for this exercise, as can a variety of squat machines.

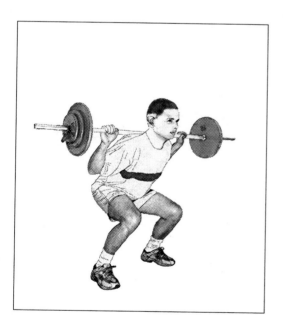 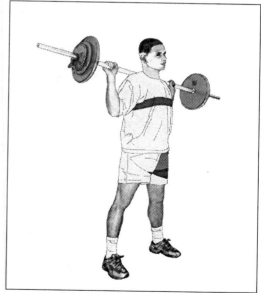

Leg Press

Muscles trained: Hips, quadriceps, buttocks, and hamstrings

Exercise type: Multi-joint

Movement execution: Seated in a leg press machine, place your feet near the top of the foot piece, with your toes pointed slightly outward and your legs at approximately shoulder-width. Unlock the weight and bend at the knees, lowering the resistance as far as is comfortable. Press the weight back up through your heels to just short of the knees-locked position.

Training tips and variations: It is suggested that you do not lock your knees at the top of the leg press. This strategy allows for maximum tension on the thighs throughout the movement. The leg press can be performed one leg at a time for variety. Many different types of leg press machines are available for use. The same training principles apply to all.

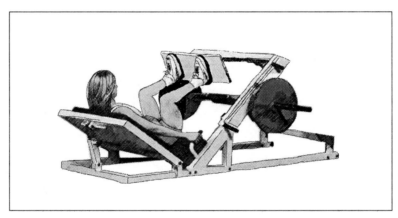

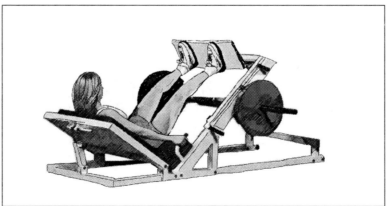

Lunge

Muscles trained: Hips, buttocks, quadriceps, hamstrings, and calves

Exercise type: Multi-joint

Movement execution: Standing upright and holding a barbell across your shoulders behind your neck, step forward, bend at the knees, and bring your rear knee close to the floor. Then, proceed by driving yourself powerfully back up to the standing position.

Training tips and variations: Lunges can be executed by alternating legs every repetition or by performing separate sets for each leg. Some trainers even prefer to walk forward for the required number of repetitions (steps), reverse course, and repeat the pattern in the opposite direction. Lunges can also be executed while holding dumbbells at your sides.

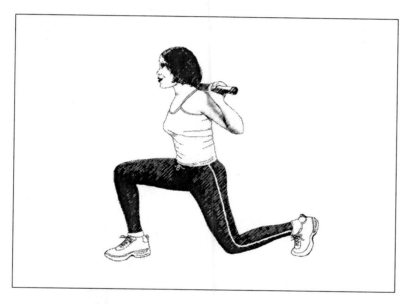

Straight-Legged Dead Lift

Muscles trained: Hamstrings and lower back

Exercise type: Multi-joint

Movement execution: While standing, take hold of a barbell with an underhand, shoulder-width grip and let the resistance hang down at arms length. Keeping your legs straight without locking your knees, bend at the waist with your back flat and your arms extended. Pause momentarily when your torso is approximately parallel to the floor and then straighten up slowly to the standing position.

Training tips and variations: It is best to perform straight-legged dead lifts in a deliberate manner, especially when incorporating heavy weights. Advanced Phase 3 athletes can execute this exercise while standing on a raised box or step in order to increase flexibility and upper hamstring involvement. Phase 1 youngsters will perform this movement with two light dumbbells in lieu of a barbell. An overhand grip can also be used for this exercise.

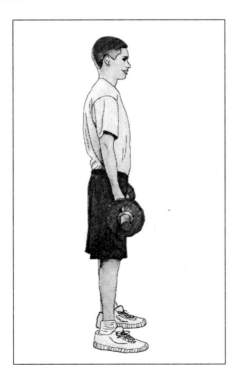 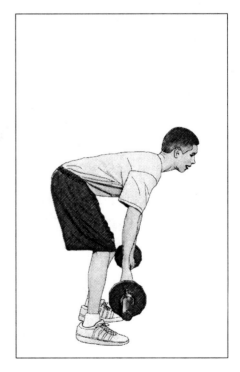

Front Squat

Muscles trained: Quadriceps, hips, buttocks, hamstrings, and lower back

Exercise type: Multi-joint

Movement execution: Place a loaded barbell at chest height on a weight rack. Step under the rack and position the bar across the front of your shoulders with your hands balancing the resistance. Your elbows should be rotated so that they are ahead of the bar. Step away from the rack and proceed to bend your knees, keeping your head up and your back straight, and lower yourself until your upper legs are just below parallel to the floor. Pause briefly and explode upward to the standing position.

Training tips and variations: Some trainers prefer to cross their arms in front of their shoulders with their hands placed on top of the bar when executing front squats. This exercise can be performed with dumbbells or on a variety of exercise machines.

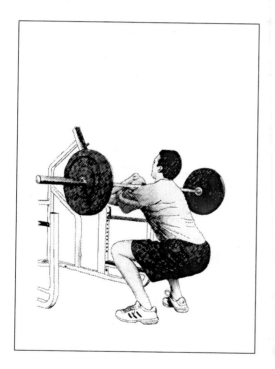
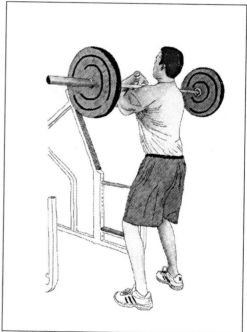

Weighted Step-Up

Muscles trained: Hips, quadriceps, buttocks, hamstrings, and calves

Exercise type: Multi-joint

Movement execution: With a barbell resting across your shoulders and your hands balancing the resistance, step up on to a box or step (the height of the box/step will depend on the youngster's stature and strength) as if climbing stairs. Pause at the top with your legs straight, and then step down carefully back to the floor.

Training tips and variations: Step-ups can be performed either by alternating legs every repetition or by executing one complete set with your left leg followed by one complete set with your right leg. Phase 1 youngsters will perform this exercise holding two light dumbbells at their sides.

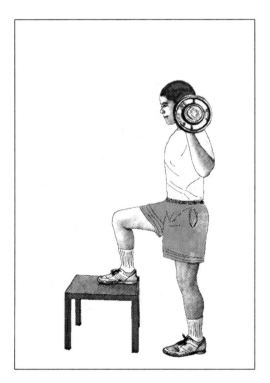 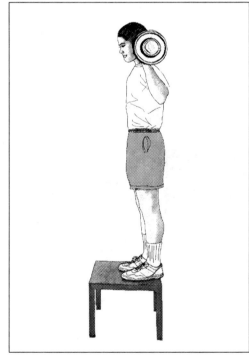

Leg Extension

Muscles trained: Quadriceps

Exercise type: Single-joint

Movement execution: Using a leg-extension machine, sit and anchor your feet under the cushions. Proceed to extend your lower legs up as high as possible and hold for a count. Lower the weight under control to the starting position.

Training tips and variations: Leg extensions can be executed one leg at a time for variety.

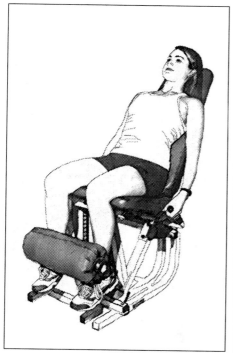 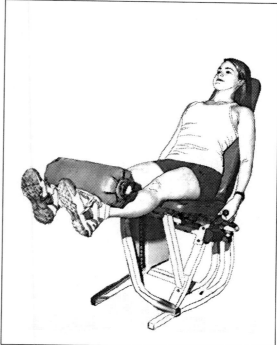

Leg Curl

Muscles trained: Hamstrings

Exercise type: Single-joint

Movement execution: Lying on your stomach on a leg-curl machine, place your heels under the pads. Using your hamstring muscles, pull your heels up as close as possible to your buttocks, while keeping your body flat on the machine. Pause for a count at the top and slowly lower the resistance back to the starting position.

Training tips and variations: Leg curls can be performed one leg at a time for variety. In addition to conventional leg-curl machines, some gyms and fitness centers have equipment that allows trainers to isolate one leg from a standing position.

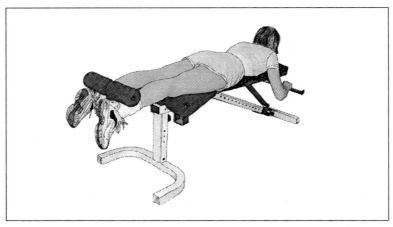

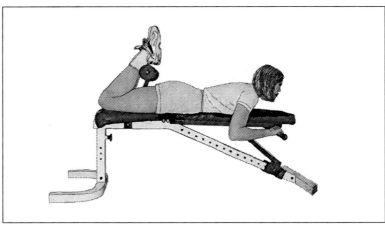

Standing Calve Raise

Muscles trained: Calves

Exercise type: Single-joint

Movement execution: Stand with your toes on a block or step with an appropriately-weighted barbell resting across your shoulders. Your hands will hold the resistance in place. Proceed by lowering your heels as far as you can toward the ground, maintaining slightly-flexed knees throughout. When you reach the fully-stretched position, come back up on your toes as high as possible.

Training tips and variations: Younger athletes (Phase 1) should perform standing calve raises with just their body weight until strength levels improve. Numerous standing calve raise machines are also available for use. The same training principles apply to all.

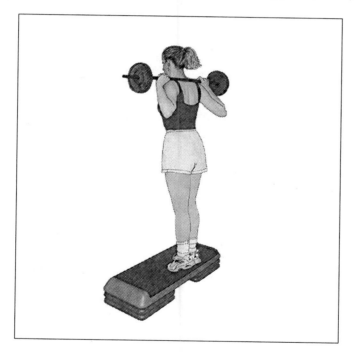

Push Press

Muscles trained: Upper chest, anterior deltoids, quadriceps, hips, lower back, and triceps

Exercise type: Combination

Movement execution: From a standing position, grab hold of a barbell off a chest-high rack with a shoulder-width grip and rest it on your upper chest just below your neck. Start by bending your knees approximately halfway to parallel and then simultaneously straighten your legs and push the weight straight up overhead. Lower the resistance slowly to the starting position.

Training tips and variations: During the positive (lifting) phase of the push press, make sure to keep your body positioned under the weight. Dumbbells can be substituted for a barbell for variety.

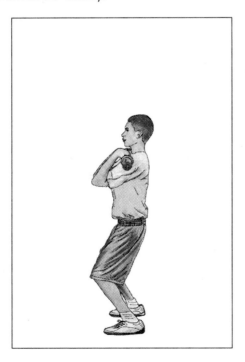 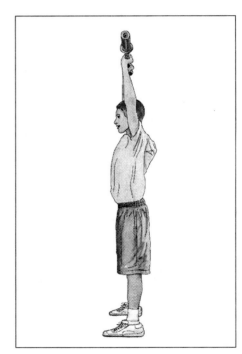

Dead Lift

Muscles trained: Hips, lower back, hamstrings, buttocks, quadriceps, entire shoulder girdle, and forearms

Exercise type: Combination

Movement execution: With feet spread slightly wider than hip-width apart, position yourself in front of a loaded barbell with your toes just inside the bar. Proceed to bend at the knees and grasp the bar with a slightly wider than shoulder width, overhand (palms facing the body) grip. Your shoulders should be in line with the bar, your elbows almost locked, your head up, and your back straight. From there, straighten the knees and lift the bar to knee height. Once the bar reaches the knees, straighten the knees, hips, and back and rest the bar on the thighs. Lower the bar carefully to the ground and repeat.

Training tips and variations: During dead lift execution, the bar can be gripped with palms facing away from the body or by having one palm facing in and one facing out. Dumbbells (as well as a variety of machines) can be used for this movement.

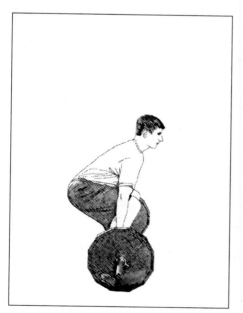 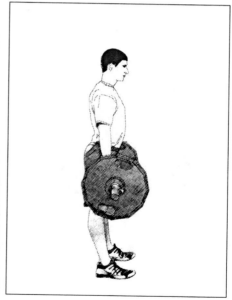

High Pull

Muscles trained: Hips, quadriceps, lower back, calves, trapezius, medial deltoids, posterior deltoids, biceps, and forearms

Exercise type: Combination

Movement execution: With an overhand, shoulder-width grip, grab a loaded barbell off a waist-high rack and position it on your lower thighs just above your knees. Your back should be flat, your head straight, your knees flexed, and your feet hip-width apart. Proceed to simultaneously raise your calves and explosively move the resistance upward as fast as possible by pulling with your arms and shrugging with your shoulders until the bar is just below your chin. The bar should remain close to your body throughout the upward movement. Lower the weight to the starting position and repeat in rapid-fire fashion.

Training tips and variations: Dumbbells can be used in place of a barbell for high pulls; however, the barbell version is far superior for strength and power development and should be used for the majority of high pull sets.

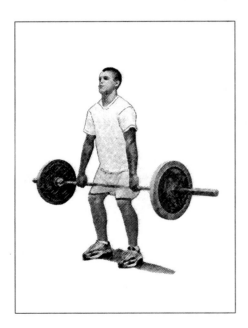 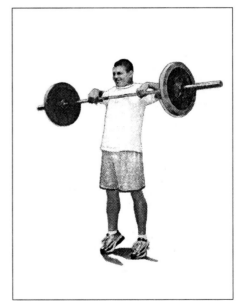

Hang Clean

Muscles trained: Hips, quadriceps, lower back, calves, anterior deltoids, medial deltoids, trapezius, forearms, and biceps

Exercise type: Combination

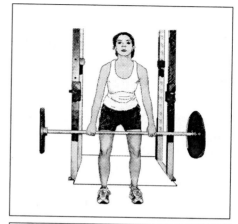

Movement execution: Assume same hand position (overhand, shoulder-width grip) and starting position (bar resting on your lower thighs) as you would when executing a high pull. Your back should be flat, your head straight, your knees flexed, and your feet at hip-width apart. Proceed to extend your hips up and slightly forward, moving on to the balls of your feet while shrugging your shoulders. From there, move under the bar, elevating your feet momentarily, and, while rotating your elbows, receive the bar on your anterior (front) deltoids. Make sure your knees and hips are sufficiently bent to absorb the resistance.

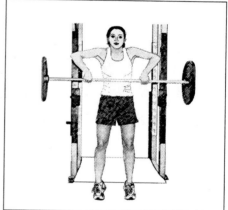

Training tips and variations: All young athletes, regardless of their experience in the weight room, should perfect hang clean form before attempting to lift heavy weights. Dumbbells can be used as a substitute for a barbell in this exercise; however, as with high pulls, the barbell version is much more effective and should be incorporated for the majority of hang clean sets.

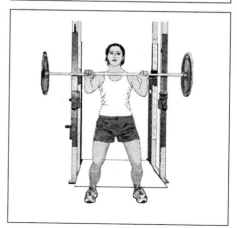

Explosive Squat

Muscles trained: Hips, quadriceps, buttocks, lower back, hamstrings, and calves

Exercise type: Combination

Movement execution: As with conventional squats, stand with your feet approximately shoulder-width apart and toes pointed slightly outward and rest a loaded barbell across your shoulders. With your hands balancing the resistance, bend your knees as if attempting to sit in a chair and lower yourself down so that your thighs are just below parallel to the floor. Keeping your head up and your back straight, explode powerfully up to the standing position, ending as high as possible on your toes. Lower to the flatfooted position, pause briefly, and repeat.

Training tips and variations: Although explosive squats are designed to be performed at a high rate of speed, it is still imperative that proper lifting form be adhered to. Dumbbells can be substituted for a barbell in this movement for variety.

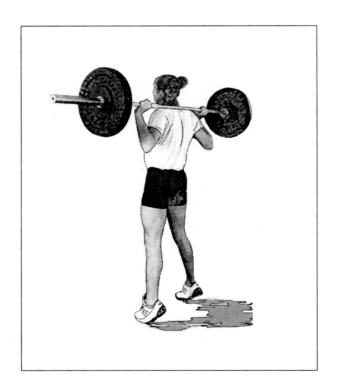

8

Youth Strength Training Program Parameters and Workouts

This chapter will help youth coaches, trainers, program administrators, and interested parents to organize and prescribe phase-appropriate strength-training programs for the young athletes under their auspices. The chapter begins each phase-specific section with program parameters and follows with a series of sample workouts that will allow youngsters of all ages to build strength in a safe, progressive, and performance-enhancing manner.

Phase 1 Strength Program

Program Parameters

- *Type of workout*: Full-body
- *Workouts per week*: Two to three
- *Total sets per workout*: 14 to 16 (not including sets for the mid-section)
- *Repetitions per set*: 15 to 20 (does not apply to abdominal training)
- *Rest between sets*: Up to two minutes
- *Training load*: Light
- *Workout duration*: 30 to 35 minutes
- *Supervision requirements*: Full-time adult supervision
- *Appropriate exercises/equipment*: Body weight, elastic bands, selected machines, dumbbells, and medicine balls
- *Training breaks per year*: Three evenly spaced training breaks of 10 to 14 days in duration
- *Emphasis*: Fun, learning proper exercise form, strength base building, weight room etiquette (no horseplay), and concentration

Tables 8-1 through 8-6 illustrate sample Phase 1 strength workouts.

Exercise	Sets and Repetitions
Body Weight Squat	3 x 20
Push-Up	3 x 15
Inverted Chin-Up	3 x 15
DB Shoulder Press	2 x 15
Elastic Band Kick-Back	1 x 20
Hammer Curl	1 x 20
Bench Crunch	3 x 15

Table 8-1. Sample Phase 1 strength workout

Exercise	Sets and Repetitions
Body Weight Step-Up	3 x 15 (each leg)
DB Incline Press	3 x 15
Pull-Down	3 x 15
Elastic Band Upright Row	2 x 15
Bench Dip	2 x 15
Calve Raise	1 x 20
Dumbbell Curl	1 x 15
Hip-Up	3 x 15

Table 8-2. Sample Phase 1 strength workout

Exercise	Sets and Repetitions
Leg Press	3 x 20
Leg Curl	2 x 20
Gravitron Chin-Up	3 x 20
DB Bench Press	3 x 15
DB Lateral Raise	2 x 15
DB Preacher Curl	1 x 15
Triceps Press-Down	1 x 15
Straight Leg Toe Touch	3 x 20

Table 8-3. Sample Phase 1 strength workout

Exercise	Sets and Repetitions
Wall Slide	3 x 20
DB Row	3 x 15
Gravitron Dip	2 x 20
DB Bent Lateral Raise	2 x 15
Elastic Band Curl	2 x 15
Lying DB Extension	2 x 15
Bicycle Sit-Up	3 x 20

Table 8-4. Sample Phase 1 strength workout

Exercise	Sets and Repetitions
DB Lunge	3 x 20
Good Morning (Med Ball)	2 x 20
Bar Push-Up	3 x 15
DB Shoulder Press	2 x 15
Seated Cable Row	3 x 15
Seated DB Triceps Ext.	2 x 15
Wrist Roller	1 x 20
Navy Seal Kicks	3 x 20

Table 8-5. Sample Phase 1 strength workout

Exercise	Sets and Repetitions
DB Dead Lift	3 x 15
Standing Calve Raise	3 x 20
Assisted Chin-Up	3 x 15
Incline DB Press	3 x 15
DB Kick-Back	2 x 15
Incline DB Curl	2 x 15
Ball Twist	3 x 20

Table 8-6. Sample Phase 1 strength workout

Phase 2 Strength Program

Program Parameters

- *Type of workout*: Full-body
- *Workouts per week*: Three
- *Total sets per workouts*: 16 to 20 (not including sets for the mid-section)
- *Repetitions per set*: 12 to 15 (does not apply to abdominal training)
- *Rest between sets*: Up to two minutes
- *Training load*: Light/Medium
- *Workout duration*: 35 to 45 minutes
- *Supervision requirements*: Full-time adult supervision
- *Appropriate exercises/equipment*: Body weight, short barbells, elastic bands, selected machines, dumbbells, and medicine balls
- *Training breaks per year*: Three evenly-spaced training breaks of seven to 10 days in duration
- *Emphasis*: Fun, learning more complicated strength movements, strength progression, confidence building, and training discipline

Tables 8-7 through 8-12 illustrate sample Phase 2 workouts.

Exercise	Sets and Repetitions
Squat	1 x 15, 2 x 12, 1 x 15
SL Dead Lift	1 x 15, 1 x 12, 1 x 15
Pull-Down	1 x 15, 1 x 12, 1 x 15
Bench Press	1 x 15, 1 x 12, 1 x 15
Upright Row	3 x 12
Triceps Press-Down	2 x 15
DB Curl	2 x 15
Bench Crunch	2 x 25
Navy Seal Kicks	2 x 25

Table 8-7. Sample Phase 2 strength workout

Exercise	Sets and Repetitions
Leg Press	1 x 15, 2 x 12, 1 x 15
Leg Curl	2 x 12
Calve Raise	2 x 15
Incline DB Press	1 x 15, 1 x 12, 1 x 15
DB Row	1 x 15, 1 x 12, 1 x 15
Floor Back Raise	2 x 15
Assisted Dip	2 x 15
Barbell Curl	2 x 12
Ball Twist	2 x 25
Hanging Leg Raise	2 x 15

Table 8-8. Sample Phase 2 strength workout

Exercise	Sets and Repetitions
Weighted Step-Up	1 x 15, 2 x 12, 1 x 15
Prone Hyper-Extension	3 x 15
Gravitron Chin-Up	1 x 15, 2 x 12, 1 x 15
Push-Up	1 x 15, 1 x 12, 1 x 15
DB Shoulder Press	1 x 15, 1 x 12, 1 x 15
Lying Triceps Extension	2 x 12
Hammer Curl	2 x 12
Hip-Up	4 x 20

Table 8-9. Sample Phase 2 strength workout

Exercise	Sets and Repetitions
Front Squat	1 x 15, 2 x 12, 1 x 15
Dead Lift	4 x 12
Reverse Back Raise	3 x 15
Seated Cable Row	2 x 15
Barbell Incline Press	2 x 12
Bent Lateral Raise	2 x 15
Preacher Curl	1 x 15
DB Kick-Back	1 x 15
Straight Leg Toe Touch	2 x 25
Bicycle Sit-Up	2 x 25

Table 8-10. Sample Phase 2 strength workout

Exercise	Sets and Repetitions
Dead Lift	1 x 15, 2 x 12, 1 x 15
Leg Extension	2 x 15
Good Morning	3 x 15
Bench Press	1 x 15, 1 x 12, 1 x 15
Pull-Down	1 x 15, 1 x 12, 1 x 15
Upright Row	1 x 15, 1 x 12, 1 x 15
Bench Dip	1 x 15
Incline DB Curl	1 x 15
Bench Crunch	3 x 25
Ball Twist	2 x 20

Table 8-11. Sample Phase 2 strength workout

Exercise	Sets and Repetitions
Lunge	3 x 15
SL Dead Lift	3 x 15
Incline Press	3 x 12
DB Row	3 x 12
Internal Rotation	2 x 15
External Rotation	2 x 15
Seated Triceps Ext.	1 x 15
Barbell Curl	1 x 15
Calve Raise	2 x 15
Hanging Leg Raise	3 x 20

Table 8-12. Sample Phase 2 strength workout

Phase 3 Strength Program

Program Parameters

- *Type of workout*: Full-body and split routine
- *Workouts per week*: Three to four
- *Total sets per workout*: 18 to 22 (not including sets for the mid-section)
- *Repetitions per set*: 6 to 12 (does not apply to abdominal training)
- *Rest between sets*: From a few seconds, as is the case when employing super sets, to up to three minutes when executing heavy multi-joint or combination lifts.
- *Training load*: Medium/Heavy
- *Workout duration*: 45 to 60 minutes
- *Supervision requirements*: Experienced Phase 3 lifters can workout together without direct supervision. However, it is still preferred that an experienced strength and conditioning specialist be on hand for all strength workouts if possible.
- *Appropriate exercises/equipment*: Body weight, barbells, elastic bands, machines, dumbbells, and medicine balls
- *Training breaks per year*: Two seven to 10 day training breaks every six months
- *Emphasis*: Satisfaction, learning and incorporating combination movements, developing sports specific/functional strength, increasing muscle size, developing an intuitive feel for strength training, and self-motivation

Tables 8-13 through 8-20 illustrate sample Phase 3 strength workouts.

Exercise	Sets and Repetitions
Machine Explosive Squat	1 x 12, 2 x 8, 1 x 10
Weighted Step-Up	1 x 12, 1 x 6, 1 x 8
Good Morning	2 x 10
Chin-Up	1 x 10, 1 x 6, 1 x 8
Dip	3 x 10
Lateral Raise	2 x 12
Preacher Curl	2 x 10
Triceps Press-Down	2 x 10
Hip-Up	3 x 25
Bicycle Sit-Up	3 x 50

Table 8-13. Sample Phase 3 full-body workout

Exercise	Sets and Repetitions
Hang Clean	1 x 12, 1 x 10, 1 x 8, 1 x 10
Bench Press	1 x 10, 1 x 8, 1 x 6, 1 x 8
Push Press	1 x 10, 1 x 8, 1 x 10
Seated Cable Row	1 x 12, 1 x 8, 1 x 10
Leg Extension	2 x 12
Leg Curl	2 x 12
Hammer Curl	2 x 10
Bench Dip	1 x 12
Straight Leg Toe Touch	3 x 50
Ball Twist (Med Ball)	2 x 25

Table 8-14. Sample Phase 3 full-body workout

Exercise	Sets and Repetitions
Front Squat	1 x 12, 1 x 8, 1 x 6, 1 x 10
SL Dead Lift	3 x 10
High Pull	1 x 10, 1 x 6, 1 x 8
Weighted Dip	1 x 12, 1 x 8, 1 x 10
Pull-Down	1 x 12, 1 x 8, 1 x 10
Barbell Curl	2 x 10
Lying Triceps	2 x 8
Bench Crunch	3 x 50
Hanging Leg Raise	3 x 25

Table 8-15. Sample Phase 3 full-body workout

Exercise	Sets and Repetitions
Leg Press	1 x 12, 1 x 8, 1 x 6, 1 x 10
Lunge	2 x 10
DB Row	1 x 10, 1 x 6, 1 x 8
Incline DB Press	1 x 10, 1 x 6, 1 x 8
Upright Row	1 x 10, 1 x 6, 1 x 6
Preacher Curl	2 x 10
Seated Triceps Press	2 x 10
Calve Raise	2 x 12
Wrist Roller	1 x 12
Straight-Leg Toe Touch	3 x 50
Ball Twist (Med Ball)	3 x 30

Table 8-16. Sample Phase 3 full-body workout

Exercise	Sets and Repetitions
Squat	1 x 12, 1 x 8, 2 x 6, 1 x 10
Dead Lift	1 x 12, 2 x 6, 1 x 10
Prone Hyper-Extension	3 x 12
Leg Extension	3 x 12
Leg Curl	3 x 10
Calve Raise	2 x 12
Bicycle Sit-Up	3 x 60
Hip-Up	3 x 50

Table 8-17. Sample Phase 3 lower body/core split workout

Exercise	Sets and Repetitions
Front Squat	1 x 12, 1 x 8, 2 x 6, 1 x 10
Weighted Step-Up	3 x 10
SL Dead Lift	4 x 8
Reverse Back Raise	3 x 12
Weighted Wall Slide	3 x 10
Calve Raise	3 x 10
Weighted Bench Crunch	3 x 20
Hanging Leg Raise	3 x 25

Table 8-18. Sample Phase 3 lower body/core split workout

Exercise	Sets and Repetitions
Hang Clean	1 x 12, 1 x 10, 1 x 6, 1 x 8
Chin-Up	1 x 12, 2 x 10, 1 x 12
Barbell Incline Press	1 x 10, 1 x 8, 1 x 6, 1 x 10
Seated Cable Row	1 x 12, 2 x 8, 1 x 10
Bent Lateral Raise	2 x 12
Cable Cross-Over	2 x 12
Triceps Press-Down	1 x 10
Incline DB Curl	1 x 10
Straight Leg Toe Touch	3 x 50
Ball Twist (Med Ball)	3 x 25

Table 8-19. Sample Phase 3 upper body/mid-section split workout

Exercise	Sets and Repetitions
Bench Press	1 x 10, 1 x 8, 2 x 6, 1 x 10
Pull-Down	1 x 12, 2 x 8, 1 x 10
High Pull	4 x 6
DB Shoulder Press	3 x 8
Weighted Dip	2 x 6
Preacher Curl	2 x 10
DB Kick-Back	2 x 12
Hip-Up	4 x 35

Table 8-20. Sample Phase 3 upper body/mid-section split workout

9

Balance Training

Good balance is a prerequisite for success in any sport. It matters not if a youngster is swinging a golf club, punting a football, or throwing a javelin, sound body balance must first be achieved prior to execution or the desired result will not occur. In fact, superior balance is the one trait that is inherent to every great athlete. Think about for a second. Some extraordinarily successful athletes do not possess outstanding speed or quickness. Others are short on strength and power. Still others want for flexibility or endurance. None, however, lack above-average balance.

Balance is also the first component of athleticism that young athletes should master. Once solid balance skills are shown, other facets (speed, agility, explosiveness, etc.) can be trained and developed to the fullest. Youth coaches and program directors who work regularly with young athletes should be acutely aware of this "balance first" principle and arrange training programs accordingly.

Parameters of Balance Training

While some young athletes have naturally better balance than others, this attribute can be improved significantly through proper training. Direct balance training is relatively new to the sports strength and conditioning field, and even many seasoned fitness professionals don't include it in their training repertoires. The workouts consist of a series of mostly unilateral exercises (exercises performed on one leg) designed to position the athlete in unstable positions, thus forcing him to acclimate or lose balance. As acclamation improves, so does balance. In addition, this type of training builds substantial strength in areas of the lower body that are rarely stimulated when executing conventional leg-strength exercises (squats, leg presses, leg extensions, etc.).

Balance training sessions will be reasonably short in duration, 15 to 20 minutes at most, and can be combined with virtually any conditioning discipline. Many find it convenient to combine balance training with either agility, explosiveness, speed, or lower body strength training, as all incorporate the same muscle groups. Some advanced youngsters may want to include a variety of de-stabilizing equipment such as foam balance pads, balance boards, and BOSU balls into their balance workouts in order to increase intensity and further balance skills.

One footnote before moving on: balance exercises are much more difficult than they appear. Even the simplest movements may prove tough for some at the beginning. Therefore, it is extremely important that youngsters not get frustrated if their initial attempts meet with futility. After a brief description of balance training equipment, a schedule description for youth balance training is put forth in the following sections.

Equipment

Athletic tape. Tape is used as a marker for line touch drills. Any type of athletic tape will suffice as long as the color contrasts with the training surface.

Medicine balls. Medicine balls will be used in a variety of balance exercises from floor pick-ups to twisting throws and catches. The weight of the ball will depend on the particular exercise and the size and strength of the youngster involved.

Balance pad. A balance pad is simply a foam mat that causes an athlete's feet to sink into the cushion, thus creating a small degree of instability. This piece of equipment is great for acclimating young Phase 1 athletes to an unstable environment.

Polyvinyl balance beams. These beams (eight feet long, four inches wide, and approximately two inches thick) allow youngsters to safely simulate gymnastic balance beam training.

Balance boards. A variety of balance boards are available for youngsters to incorporate into their balance workouts. Most consist of a single platform with a fulcrum (or fulcrums) underneath that creates an unstable environment forcing practitioners to constantly adjust to maintain balance. Some state of the art balance boards move in three axes for greater instability. Before a balance board is used, youngsters must first master all ground-based balance exercises.

BOSU ball. A BOSU ball is a soft, half moon shaped ball that provides an extremely unstable standing environment. Training balance on a BOSU ball is very challenging, and should only be engaged in by advanced Phase 3 youngsters. This equipment is now featured at most public fitness facilities.

Footwear. Many strength and conditioning specialists recommend that balance training be performed barefoot. They feel that this approach will strengthen the feet, ankles, and lower legs to a greater degree. Of course, if balance training on a rough surface or while nursing any type of lower leg or foot injury, wearing conventional basketball or cross-training footwear is suggested.

Schedule Description

Program Length

A balance-training program for young athletes is a year-round endeavor. Unlike explosiveness, speed, and agility training, direct balance work involves no impact to the ground, making it easy on the joints with a very low risk of injury.

Number of Workouts Per Week

Two direct balance workouts per week performed on a year-round basis are suggested for all phases of development.

Sets and Repetitions

Phase 1: sets = six to eight, repetition range = eight to 10.
Phase 2: sets = eight to 10, repetition range = 10 to 12
Phase 3: sets = 10 to 12, repetition range = 12 to 16

Usually sets of balance training will be spread among three to five different exercises. Please note: in balance training terminology, one set will include performing the given exercise on each leg.

Rest Between Sets

The rest between sets of balance exercises will range from 30 to 60 seconds depending on the intensity of the movement and the capabilities of the young practitioners. For example, a set of single leg stands will require much less recovery time than will a set of medicine ball pick-ups performed standing on a BOSU ball.

Workout Duration

Most balance workouts can be performed in less than 20 minutes.

Balance Exercises

Single-leg stand. This simple exercise entails standing erect on one leg with your knee slightly flexed for 30 to 60 seconds. The raised leg should be bent at the knee and positioned behind your body approximately parallel to the floor. To increase difficulty, try this exercise with eyes closed. Single-leg stands are best performed on a soft surface such as a balance pad.

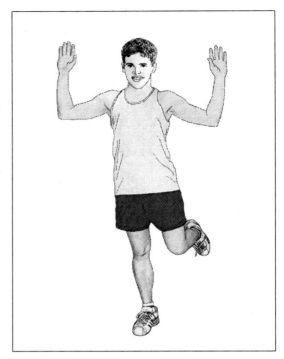

Curb walk. Curb walks resemble what a gymnast would do on a balance beam—minus the flips and cartwheels of course. Once an appropriately-sized curb is located (polyvinyl balance beams can also be used), proceed to step one foot in front of the other without falling off. The distance of the walk can vary from a few steps to 10 yards or more depending on proficiency and available landscape. In order to increase the difficulty of this exercise, youngsters can carry light dumbbells in each hand during execution.

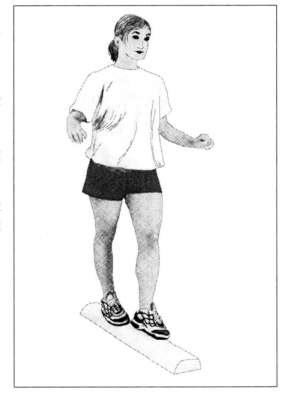

Line touch. Place a strip of athletic tape on the floor in front of you. Stand on one leg where the tape begins and, with your back straight, proceed to bend at the hips, knee, and ankle, reaching as far as you can with the hand that correlates with the raised leg and touch the tape. Make sure to mark your results from week to week to check progress.

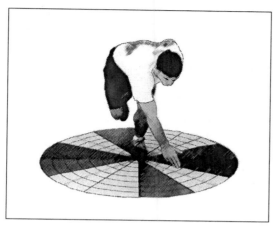

One-legged medicine ball chest pass and catch. Stand as you would during single leg stands holding an appropriately weighted medicine ball with two hands at chest height. Your elbows should be bent so that the ball is positioned a few inches from your body. Remaining on one leg throughout, toss the ball back and forth with a partner standing six to eight yards directly in front of you. Continue for the required number of repetitions. Switch standing legs and repeat. Phase 1 youngsters may want to use a basketball, soccer ball, or volleyball in lieu of a medicine ball for this drill until the necessary strength is developed. Advanced young athletes can incorporate a balance board or some other unstable standing surface to increase difficulty.

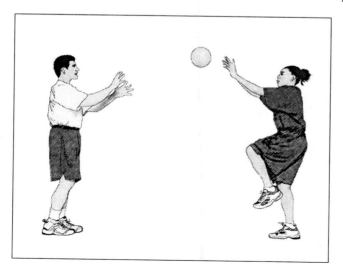

Ball pick-up. Place a basketball, volleyball, or appropriately-weighted medicine ball approximately two to three feet in front of you. Begin by standing on one leg with your knee slightly flexed. Then, bend forward at the hips, knee, and ankle and with both hands grab the ball from the floor and rise up to the standing position. The ball can either be brought up to the mid-section or (to increase difficulty) overhead. After completing each repetition, hand the ball to a coach or training partner and have him place it back on the floor. To increase difficulty, execute the exercise on an unstable surface such as a BOSU ball or balance board and/or have your coach/training partner place the ball in different, more challenging positions (left, right, farther away, etc.).

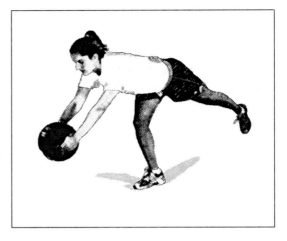

Around the world. Standing on your right leg with your hips, knee, and ankle slightly flexed, move either a volleyball, basketball, or appropriately weighted medicine ball as fast as possible under your knee from right to left, then back around your back from left to right. Pause briefly and reverse course (right to left around your back, left to right under your knee) and continue in this pattern for the required number of repetitions. Stand on the left leg and repeat the action. To increase difficulty, try performing this exercise on an unstable surface such as a balance pad or balance board.

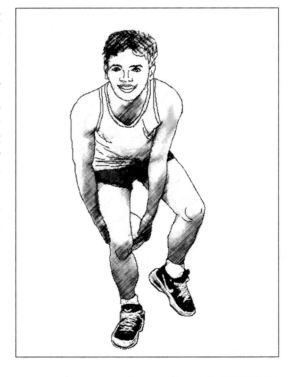

One-legged side toss and catch. Stand on one leg with your grounded knee slightly flexed. Your raised leg should be bent at the knee and placed behind your body parallel to the ground. Begin by twisting your torso as far as you can in the direction of the grounded leg and receive a passed medicine ball from your partner who will be standing six to eight feet away off your shoulder. Once the catch is secured, immediately position the ball just above waist height, eight to 12 inches from your body. From there, twist your torso as far as possible in the opposite direction, keeping your arms and grounded leg stationary throughout. Then, in a controlled but powerful manner, swing back and release the ball to your training partner. Repeat the action while standing on the opposite leg. Younger, less-advanced athletes should perform this exercise with a basketball in lieu of a medicine ball.

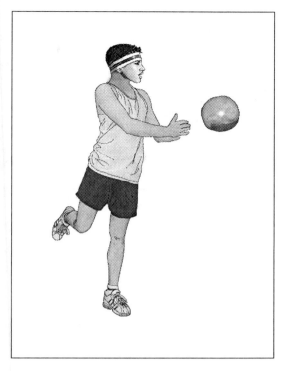

Single-leg below plane squat. Stand on one leg positioned on a step, plyometric box, or BOSU ball. Proceed by squatting down on the grounded leg until the non-grounded leg is below the plane of the standing surface. How far a young athlete lowers himself depends on individual strength, flexibility, and balance. This movement is very demanding and should only be performed by advanced Phase 2 and Phase 3 youngsters.

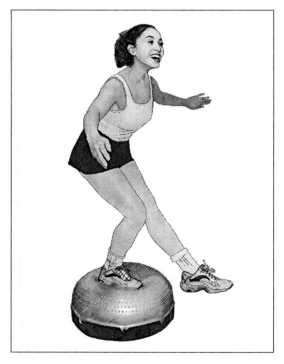

Tables 9-1 through 9-3 provide sample phase-appropriate balance workouts.

Exercise	Sets and Repetitions
Single Leg Stands	3 x 45 seconds
Curb Walks	2 x 8 (six yards each)
Line Touches	3 x 10

Table 9-1. Sample Phase 1 balance workout

Exercise	Sets and Repetitions
Curb Walks	2 x 10 (eight yards each)
Line Touches	3 x 12
Around the Worlds	3 x 10
Ball Pick-Ups (Basketball)	2 x 10

Table 9-2. Sample Phase 2 balance workout

Exercise	Sets and Repetitions
Around the Worlds	3 x 12
Ball Pick-Ups (Medicine)	3 x 14
Side Toss and Catch	3 x 12
Below Plane Squat	3 x 16

Table 9-3. Sample Phase 3 balance workout

10

Speed Training

Huge strides (no pun intended) have been made in recent years when it comes to increasing running speed. After decades where even top track coaches were staunch in their belief that speed was a strictly inherited trait (a favorite saying was, "sprinters are born, not made"), it is now universally accepted in the sports world that athletes, through proper and focused training, can increase their short distance (less than 200 meters) sprinting speed substantially.

This epiphany concerning improving running speed could not have come at a better time for aspiring young athletes. They have the opportunity, which past generations of athletes were not afforded, to learn and implement a variety of specialized speed-enhancing techniques when their bodies are most receptive to improvement. Mastering these methods early in life will allow youngsters to not only reach their full potential as sprinters, but it will enable them to use this newfound speed throughout their athletic careers (which hopefully spans many years into the future).

Three Paths for Increasing Sprinting Speed

The three basic paths for increasing sprinting speed are: physical conditioning, athletic ability, and running mechanics. Training each of these components effectively will help young athletes improve their ability to run fast. The three paths for increasing sprinting speed are explained in detail in the following sections.

Conditioning

Youngsters who hope to reach their full running speed potential must first acquire a high level of physical conditioning, which means being both aerobically and anaerobically fit in relation to their age and physical maturity and achieving an optimal athletic body weight.

Solid cardiovascular fitness will allow young athletes to train consistently hard without fatiguing, which is a prerequisite when it comes to tolerating demanding speed workouts. In short, young bodies must be up to the task physically if substantial speed increases are to take place.

Realizing individual ideal body weight speaks for itself. Not too many overweight athletes run fast. And if they do, they could surely run quite a bit faster if a proper body weight was maintained. Carrying too much poundage on the frame also increases the risk for lower body impact-related injuries such as shin splints, stress fractures, and knee cartilage tears—not to mention bringing with it numerous negative health consequences such as high blood pressure, diabetes, and heart disease.

It is not necessary that we go further into detail about specific conditioning methods here (the rest of the book does that), but youngsters of all ages must realize that in order to run as fast as their genetics will allow, attaining top shape is the first step.

Athletic Ability

Athletic ability has many definitions. For the purposes of this chapter, it will refer to the attributes of quickness, agility, flexibility, strength, balance, and explosiveness. Improving these aspects will help youngsters run faster. The quicker and more agile a young athlete is, the faster he'll reach his maximum speed (acceleration). The ability to accelerate quickly is crucial to success in most sports, and on the whole is more coveted in the athletic community than is possessing a high maximum speed. The more flexible the muscles, the better they will respond when sprinting, especially when it comes to increasing stride length—an important factor in how fast an individual runs. (Stride length is discussed in the next section on running mechanics.) A stronger lower body will enable young athletes to generate more force off the ground during the stride cycle, thus translating into more speed. Improving upper body strength also contributes to increasing running speed by allowing for more powerful arm motion. The better-balanced runner will be the more efficient runner. Increased running efficiency equals faster sprinting. Explosiveness training techniques such as plyometrics effects forceful muscular contractions, which leads to faster movement whether running, jumping, or throwing.

The great news concerning all of these athletic attributes is that they can be improved significantly by following the training programs and suggestions in this book. Focused work on enhancing athletic ability will pay great dividends when it comes time to hit the track, field, beach, or hills for speed workouts—not to mention when sprinting full-speed during sports competitions.

Running Mechanics

An important and surprisingly neglected variable in increasing sprinting speed involves improving and perfecting running mechanics. Although every individual has a unique running style, young athletes can implement numerous fundamental speed-enhancing techniques that will help them reach their ultimate sprinting potential.

The two major factors in how fast someone can run can be described in a simple equation: stride length x stride frequency = running speed. Stride length is the space covered in an individual stride. Stride frequency is the time it takes to accomplish a single stride. To become faster sprinters, youngsters must enhance their stride length by intensifying the force against the ground, while maintaining balance with their stride frequency. Powerful and efficient arm movement also must be employed. The following list details the characteristics of effective sprinting:

- During the first few strides from a stationary position, it is important to stay low. Standing up too quickly at the onset of a run will slow speed considerably.
- Once the first few yards of a sprint are covered, running in a naturally erect position is central to good sprinting technique. Many young athletes have been erroneously taught to lean forward when sprinting. This positioning will actually slow down the runner and can contribute to a loss of balance at high speeds.
- The head should be up and straight, with eyes focused toward the destination of the run.
- Arms, shoulders, and hands should be relaxed when sprinting. Many young athletes have a tendency to keep their upper bodies rigid when running at top speed. Remember, for youngsters to reach their sprinting potential, they must always remain relaxed.
- The push-off leg should always end up completely extended during the stride cycle.
- Overstriding should be avoided. Increasing stride length in unnatural fashion by forcing the lead foot to land too far ahead of the body will hinder sprinting speed.
- Arm action should come from the shoulders when sprinting. During the upswing, hands should reach just in front of the chin and slightly inside the shoulders. On the downswing, hands should reach no further back than the hips.
- Artificially increasing stride frequency by attempting to move the legs too quickly, will make the runner move fast but mostly in one place—not very helpful when beating out an infield hit, sprinting back on defense in a basketball game, or running a pass pattern in football.
- The elbows should be kept at a 90-degree angle, forcing all arm action to stay close to the body. If the arms are too far from the torso when sprinting, it will disrupt stride rhythm.
- The torso should remain mostly stationary when sprinting, with the shoulders squared to the destination of the run.

Like all athletic skills, sprinting properly requires repetitive practice. Youngsters should aspire to the best of their ability to follow these guidelines whenever full-speed running is required (conditioning workouts, sports-specific drills, sports competition, etc.). Additionally, it is highly recommended that young athletes seek out experienced track and/or running coaches for instruction and training. Most high school and college track programs have knowledgeable coaches on staff who are usually more than happy to share their expertise.

Specialized Drills and Techniques for Developing Speed

Young athletes will incorporate three different types of drills in their speed training: speed technique drills, resistance sprinting, and overspeed training. All three are discussed in detail in the following sections, along with a variety corresponding drills.

Speed Technique Drills

Speed technique drills, as the name suggests, are designed to improve a youngsters running form. The movements range in intensity from very light (arm swings) to reasonably high (acceleration sprints). In order to get the most out of speed technique drills, young athletes must remain focused on proper running form. With enough repetition, mind and body will synchronize, allowing correct running form to come about naturally without conscious effort.

Drill: Standing Arm Swings

Execution: Stand with your knees slightly bent and your legs shoulder width apart. Proceed to swing your arms powerfully as if you were sprinting.

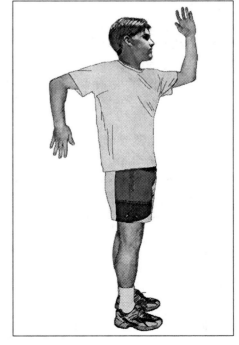

Drill: Seated Arm Swings

Execution: Sit on the floor with your legs straight out in front of you. Proceed to swing your arms powerfully as if you were sprinting.

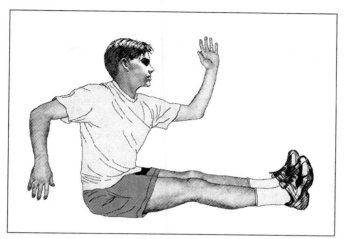

Drill: Up and Downs

Execution: Standing with a straight posture, attempt to lift one knee as high as possible while keeping the opposite leg planted firmly on the ground. Alternate legs each repetition. Arms should swing up and down naturally, as if running in place.

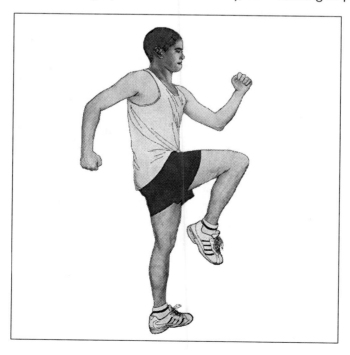

Drill: Leg Pull Through

Execution: With one leg flat on the ground, extend your other leg out in front of you. Proceed by pulling the extended leg down to the ground in a powerful, yet controlled manner. Repeat equally with both legs.

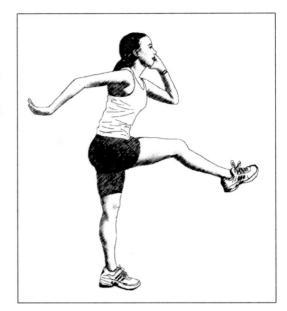

Drill: Form Strides

Execution: Stride at a medium, even pace over the course of the run, always focusing on form rather than speed. Form strides can range in distance between 50 and 200 hundred meters depending on training objective.

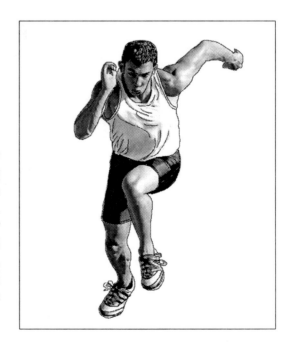

Drill: Acceleration Sprints

Execution: Begin by running at a slow pace and proceed by gradually increasing your speed over the course of the run until top speed is attained. For example, if you were engaging in a 100-meter acceleration sprint, you would commence by striding about 15 meters, accelerating for 40 meters or so, and then ramp up to an all-out sprint for the duration of the drill.

Drill: Ladder Sprints

Execution: Spread a speed ladder out over a soft, even running surface. The ladder itself will consist of 10 to 12 rungs, which have graduated spacing from shortest to longest. Proceed to sprint explosively between each rung, maintaining proper running form throughout.

Working out with a speed ladder forces the runner to take short, quick steps at the beginning of a sprint, which discourages the common problem of overstriding and allows for faster acceleration.

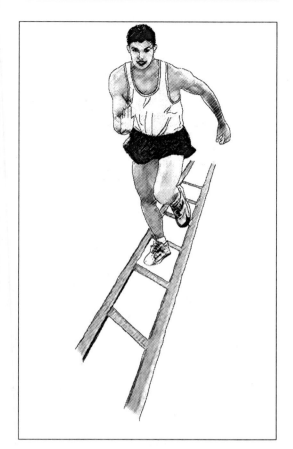

Drill: High Knee Barrier Runs

Execution: Face a line of 10 to 14 banana-step barriers, each spread approximately three feet apart. The height of the barriers can range from six to 18 inches depending on the size and athletic ability of the drill participant. Proceed to run through the line of barriers with knees high and arm motion exaggerated. When the end of the line is reached, turn 180 degrees and repeat the movement pattern. Continue for the required number of repetitions.

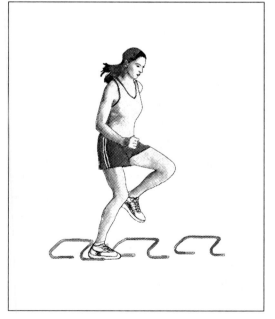

Added Resistance Sprinting

Added resistance sprinting calls for adding weight or resistance to a young athlete's frame in order to make the act of sprinting more difficult, thus facilitating increased running speed. Youngsters can accomplish this in a number of ways. The following are some of the most popular and effective of these.

Uphill sprinting. Sprinting up hills is a tried and true method of training that increases running speed. Athletes in a variety of sports including football, track, basketball, and soccer incorporate this technique in their workout regimens on a regular basis. And, unlike many other resistance sprinting disciplines, it costs nothing in terms of fancy equipment. The only requirement is an appropriate running landscape.

The hill grade for uphill sprint sessions will vary depending on the training objectives and conditioning level of the young athlete involved. As a rule, steep grades (seven- to 10-degree angles) should be utilized for short, explosive runs covering five to 15 yards or so. Flatter grades (1.5- to 3.5-degree angles) should be used for longer sprints (20 to 80 yards). Any other type of resistance equipment (i.e., weighted vest) should never be incorporated for uphill sprints. The hills themselves will provide more than enough resistance.

Weighted-vest sprinting. Sprinting while wearing a weighted vest has shown to be an effective way to improve running speed and explosiveness. However, if executed improperly, it can also be dangerous, especially for young, developing athletes. The correct (and safe) way to incorporate a weighted vest in a youngster's speed-training program is discussed as follows:

- The weight of the vest should never be heavier than eight to 10 percent of a youngster's body weight. A higher ratio of vest weight to body weight will compromise running form and increase the injury risk substantially.
- Weight should be added to the vest gradually from workout to workout as strength, speed, and conditioning improvements warrant. Even elite athletes follow this protocol, sometimes taking a half-dozen weighted-vest sprint workouts before increasing weight.
- It is imperative that young athletes incorporate proper and natural running form when engaging in weighted-vest sprint workouts. If the weight of the vest interferes with running form, the vest is too heavy and should be lightened. It is always better to perform these sessions with less weight, rather than compromising technique and risking injury by pushing it.
- Young athletes who suffer from lower back or knee problems should consider skipping this training method. The additional weight of the vest, even if it's only a small percentage of body weight, can nevertheless exacerbate existing conditions.

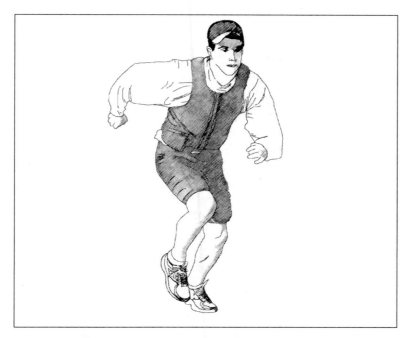

Two-person harness. Track athletes and football players frequently use the two-person harness to improve their acceleration. It features waist and shoulder straps that fasten to the runner and handles that are held by the training partner/coach during drill execution. Training with this equipment entails having one partner firmly hold the handles and attempt not to give ground while the other partner who is wearing the harness sprints straight ahead, pulling the resistance to the best of his ability. Two-person harness sprint drills are most effective for short distance runs of 10 to 20 yards.

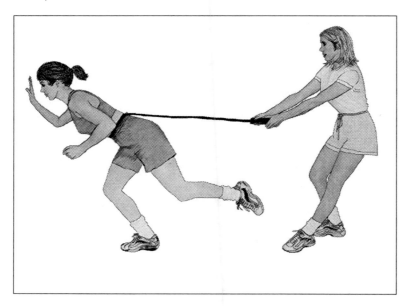

Resistance parachute. Sales of resistance parachutes have skyrocketed in recent years. Especially in the youth sports community, as the equipment's high-tech look is a magnet for the attention of youngsters. Notwithstanding their fancy appearance, resistance parachutes, if designed and used properly, do provide speed benefits.

The parachute itself is attached to the body by a waist strap. The idea then is to accelerate gradually into a full sprint, allowing the chute to catch the wind, open, and proceed to make the run more difficult. Most newer versions of the resistance parachute come with a quick release feature that allows for mid-stride release, thus promoting a sudden burst of speed that can increase stride frequency. Parachute workouts are best accomplished on a running track or on a well-manicured football or soccer field.

The biggest disadvantage of the resistance parachute (other than the cost) is durability. They are known to tangle, not open, and rip during workouts. Purchasing the equipment from a reliable manufacturer is the only defense against these frustrating malfunctions.

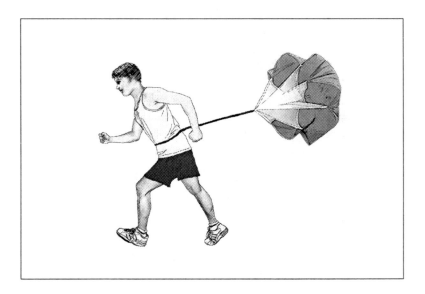

Sled pulls. Resistance sleds are used frequently by football players and are actually modeled to some extent after the old-fashion blocking sleds seen on most football practice fields. The only difference is that blocking sleds are designed to be pushed while resistance sleds are made to be pulled.

Execution is simple. Just adjust the weight of the sled (usually accomplished by adding or subtracting barbell plates), attach the shoulder/waist harness, and proceed to sprint forward explosively while remaining as low as possible.

Sled pulls are best executed on a stretch of even, low-cut grass. Uneven or rocky terrain makes the sled awkward to move and can increase the risk of injury. As with two-person harness training, this overspeed method is most effective for speed development when incorporated over short distances.

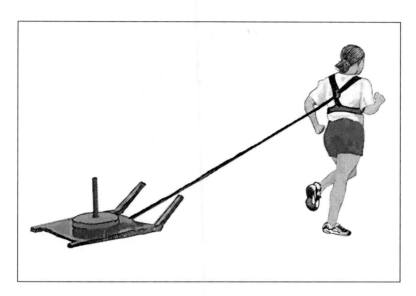

Water sprinting. Water provides natural and safe resistance, thus running in a pool is a terrific low-impact way to garner a productive sprint workout. Water treadmills are also available for use at many heath clubs, fitness centers, and university athletic facilities. This equipment allows the youngster to run on a submerged footpad against water current that can be adjusted to suit individual needs. Water sprint workouts are the only added-resistance sprinting technique appropriate for injured young athletes.

Stadium step running. Athletes in a variety of sports incorporate stadium step running in their speed-training programs. All young athletes need to perform this resistance sprinting method is access to a reasonably large sports stadium (most colleges with a football team have them). In a pinch, stairwells of office buildings, high-rise apartment complexes, or schools can be used.

What makes step running such a tremendous resistance speed workout is that the time the foot spends in the push-off phase is substantially longer than when training on level ground. This provides a greater training effect. The emphasis during these workouts should be on high knee lift. Youngsters are encouraged to explode upward from step to step to the best of their ability. Because legs will be extremely fatigued once the top of the stairs are reached, it is imperative that young athletes take great care when descending so as to avoid stumbling. Adults supervising stadium step workouts should encourage this mindful decent subsequent to every set.

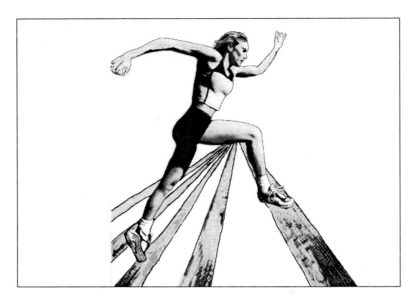

Arm motion with resistance. Resisted arm motion is an effective technique for promoting powerful arm movement during sprinting. It is performed as follows: standing with knees slightly flexed, grab hold of two reasonably light dumbbells and position them at your hips with palms facing your body. Proceed to alternately hammer curl the weight up and down, incorporating sprinting arm motion. Continue for the required number of repetitions. Small medicine balls or weighted beanbags can be substituted for dumbbells for this drill.

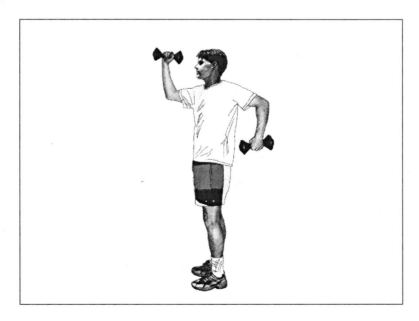

Overspeed Training

Overspeed training will enhance a young athlete's ability to run fast by increasing stride length and frequency. Similar to plyometrics (Chapter 12), this type of training forces the neuromuscular system to become accustomed to faster speeds and, therefore, enables youngsters to attain those speeds without facilitation. Overspeed training is very intense and demands complete concentration and a high level of physical conditioning. As such, while overspeed workouts are appropriate for all phases of athletic development, coaches, trainers, and program administrators should be aware of individual limitations and act accordingly in prescribing overspeed drills to youngsters. A variety of speed-promoting overspeed methods are discussed in the following sections.

Downhill sprinting. Downhill sprinting is the oldest and among the most reliable forms of overspeed training. It entails simply sprinting down an appropriately steep hill with your body balanced and your running form sound. Full concentration must be brought to all downhill sprint repetitions, or a tumble down the hill could be in the cards. The downgrade of the hill should be approximately three-degrees. Anything steeper is not advisable for young athletes, because it will compromise running form and can be dangerous. The length of the downhill stretch can range from 10 to 40 meters depending on the training objectives of the participant. No extra equipment (i.e., weighed vest) should be incorporated during downhill sessions. Young athletes must be sufficiently warmed up prior to all downhill sprinting workouts, for obvious reasons.

Towing. Towing is perhaps the most popular form of overspeed training among high-level athletes—the reason being that it works. The execution is as follows: attach the towing apparatus, which consists of strong elastic tubing and a waist belt, to the runner's body and then to a training partner or secure object such as a goal post or backstop. From there, the runner proceeds to walk backwards facing the partner/secure object for approximately 30 meters. After a brief pause, the runner begins to sprint straight ahead at full speed as the tubing snaps back and pulls him forward.

Towing workouts should always be executed on soft, even running surfaces such as well-manicured football or soccer fields, rubberized running tracks, or stretches of Astroturf or field turf. Proper running form must be maintained during towing sprints. If the youngster has trouble maintaining running form, this technique should not be used. Most well made elastic tubing will stretch five to six times its relaxed length. For safety reasons, an adult should check for any damage to the tubing prior to all towing repetitions.

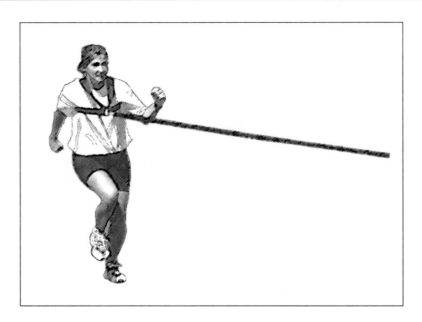

High-speed treadmill sprinting. High-speed treadmill running has become a widely used form of overspeed training throughout the sports strength and conditioning community, especially in those areas of the country and the world where the winters are not conducive to outdoor sprint workouts. It improves both stride length and frequency, and has produced speed gains for numerous athletes in a variety of sports.

This technique works best when the sprinter enters the treadmill running surface when it is already moving at a high rate of speed. Therefore, practicing getting on the belt at slower speeds is a prerequisite for all youngsters before high-speed entry is attempted. Four to six workouts of gradually increasing entry speed is suggested. It is also recommended that two adult spotters—one positioned on each side of the machine at the runner's shoulder—are on hand for all high-speed treadmill sessions. Obviously, a full-scale warm-up should be engaged in prior to these types of workouts.

Before commencing with treadmill overspeed training, coaches/trainers should have a good idea how fast in miles per hour a young athlete can run 40 yards. Once this is determined, the treadmill speed should be set at one to four miles-per-hour above maximum speed. The time/distance conversion rate for treadmill overspeed training is about 1.0 second = 10 yards. Because of the complicated entry method described in the preceding paragraphs, treadmill overspeed training is only appropriate for Phase 3 and advanced Phase 2 athletes.

High-speed stationary cycling. High-speed stationary cycling, according to some, can assist in increasing a sprinter's stride frequency during the stride cycle. Preliminary evidence seems to bear this out; however, most sports speed experts feel that this method, while marginally effective, is not nearly as helpful for increasing overall running speed as is downhill sprinting or towing. As such, high-speed stationary cycling will be used only as an adjunct to the previously mentioned overspeed techniques.

The workouts themselves will consist of one- to three-second repetitions of sprint-assisted pedaling, followed by 10 seconds or so of deceleration. To ensure total recovery, two minutes of easy pedaling at approximately 30 revolutions-per-minute should occur after the deceleration period. Three to 10 total repetitions per workout will be accomplished depending on the strength, conditioning, and goals of the young athlete.

Follow the leader. This type of overspeed training is more psychological than physiological. It is executed as follows: start by giving a training partner a five- to 10-foot head start in a sprint race. Then try to catch up with him over the course of the run. The distance of a "follow the leader" sprint can vary from 20 to 200 yards, depending on the youngster's training objectives.

The follow the leader drill is considerably less demanding from a physical standpoint than that of other overspeed methods, however, because of the pride/competition component (the determination to catch or at least gain ground on the partner), it has shown to be a fun and productive way for young athletes to increase sprinting speed.

11

Agility and Quickness Training

Agility is defined as the ability to change direction efficiently at high rates of speed. Quickness specifies how quickly an individual can move from one place to another, usually within a six-foot radius. Both of these attributes are extremely important in all movement-intensive sports such as basketball, soccer, tennis, lacrosse, and field hockey to name just a few. In fact, in many sports agility and quickness are more coveted than straight ahead running speed. Agility/quickness training is appropriate and safe for all age groups and, best of all, it's a fun and creative way to enhance athleticism and conditioning in youngsters.

Schedule Description

Agility/quickness training should be undertaken on a year-round basis. Three workouts per week are suggested when not participating in an organized sports season. During a season, two workouts every seven days or so should suffice. Agility/quickness sessions can be performed on their own, within the context of a team practice, or in combination with balance, speed or plyometric workouts. All workouts should be executed on flat, semi-soft surfaces such as even, low-cut grass, rubberized running tracks, or wood flooring; basketball/volleyball courts are preferred by many for this type of training, as their existing floor lines can be used for markers.

An almost countless number of agility/quickness drills are available to young athletes. Some of the most useful and popular are documented at the end of this chapter. However, these drills are just the tip of the iceberg as far as drill options are concerned. Therefore, coaches, trainers, and youngsters themselves should feel free to experiment with a variety of different movement patterns. Enterprising individuals may want to try their hand at designing their own drills to fit specific athletic needs.

Sets of agility/quickness drills will be short in duration (10 to 20 seconds per set on average) and are designed to be performed with all-out effort. Once movement patterns are mastered, youngsters in Phases 2 and 3 of development are encouraged to execute each set at full speed. Phase 1 athletes will put more emphasis on maintaining balance and perfecting footwork than on speed and intensity in the early stages of their agility/quickness training. However, they too will move toward full-speed execution once individual comfort levels are established. All age groups should attempt to incorporate "light feet" (soft and quick foot contacts with the ground) during all agility/quickness drills. This technique will not only help to increase foot quickness, but lessen the impact of each footfall, thus decreasing injury risk.

Equipment

One of the great things about agility/quickness training is that it requires very little in the way of equipment. However, a few items to which every young agility/quickness trainer should have access are listed in the following sections.

Agility ladder. Agility ladders are currently very popular in the sports strength and conditioning community. They include a series of flat, evenly-spaced rungs that can be spread out easily over any appropriate training surface. Most agility ladders are 10 yards long with rungs that measure approximately 16 inches in width and 18 inches in length. The most up to date equipment can be snapped apart at the midpoint, which allows for shorter distance and change of direction drills.

Cones. Cones are used to designate movement patterns in a variety of agility drills. Depending on the particular drill, the cones can range in height from a few inches to foot or more. Barriers, as long as they are made of soft plastic or rubber, can be substituted for cones for agility workouts.

Athletic tape. Athletic tape will be incorporated as markers for quick movement agility drills such as front and lateral line hops. Of course, if agility workouts are taking place on a well-lined basketball or volleyball court, the need for tape markers will be minimal.

Reaction ball. These balls are small, unevenly shaped objects that bounce in unpredictable fashion. The goal of reaction ball drills is to chase down and pick up the ball as quickly as possible.

Reaction belt. A reaction belt is an approximately five-foot long, break-free Velcro belt that attaches to the waists of two drill participants, one of whom is the movement initiator and the other the movement follower. The object of the drill is for the movement follower to keep the belt on as long as possible, ideally until the end of the drill.

Agility/quickness workout parameters are detailed in Table 11-1.

Program length:	Year-round
Drills per workout:	3 to 6
Sets per drill:	2 to 4 (Phase 1)
	4 to 6 (Phase 2)
	6 to 8 (Phase 3)
Drill duration:	10 to 30 seconds
Rest between sets:	30 to 60 seconds
Days per week:	3 days (off season)
	2 days (in-season)
Intensity:	Medium (Phase 1)
	High (Phases 2 and 3)

Table 11-1. Recommended parameters for youth agility/quickness training

Agility/Quickness Drills

A young athlete's agility/quickness training will consist of three different types of drills: quick movement, specific movement pattern, and random movement pattern. Each serves a particular athletic-enhancement purpose.

Quick movement drills entail a series of short distance hops and foot movements performed in rapid fire fashion that encourage young athletes to move their feet as fast as possible. Specific movement pattern drills include sports functional movement patterns (side shuffles, backpedals, straight short sprints, etc.). They help to develop general footwork skills and in-motion body balance. Random movement pattern drills are the most challenging of the group. Performing them regularly will advance a youngster's ability to change direction quickly, start and stop efficiently, and react to unplanned situations as he would during a sports competition. Some drills in this section will also require the use of hand-eye coordination skills.

Generally speaking, agility/quickness training workouts for youngsters will feature an equal number of each of the previously mentioned drill types. However, exceptions can be made relative to age, physical maturity, and practitioner experience. For example, some Phase 3 athletes may want to add a few extra sets of random movement pattern drills to their agility workouts from time to time. On the other hand, slower developing Phase 1 children are best served focusing on perfecting quick movement and specific movement pattern drill execution before moving onto the more complicated random movements.

Quick Movement Drills

Drill: Front Line Hops

Execution: Stand facing a line with your feet close together and your knees slightly bent. On command, hop back and forth over the line as fast as possible. Continue for the required time.

Drill: Lateral Line Hops

Execution: Stand parallel to a line with your feet close together and your knees slightly bent. On command, hop back and forth laterally over the line as fast as possible. Continue for the required time.

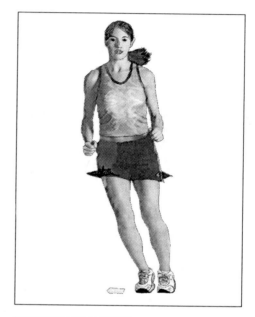

Drill: Four Way Box Hops

Execution: Place two pieces of athletic tape in a box shape in front of you. Proceed to hop as quickly as possible from one quadrant to the other in one direction for the required time. After an appropriate rest interval, reverse course and repeat.

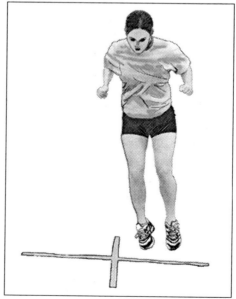

Drill: One Leg Hops Series

Execution: Perform all the preceding drills on one leg.

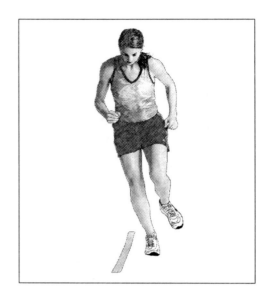

Drill: Front In and Outs

Execution: Begin by facing the front of an agility ladder. On "go," proceed to step into the first rung of the ladder with your right foot, followed immediately by stepping into the same rung with your left foot. Once the left foot lands, quickly step outside of the ladder with your right foot. From there, shift your weight through the hips and step forward with your left foot to the second rung. Once the left foot lands, immediately step back into the second rung with your right foot. Proceed to step out of ladder with your left foot and then shift your weight through the hips and step forward with your right foot into the third run. Continue in this sequence to the end of the ladder. Repeat for the required number of repetitions.

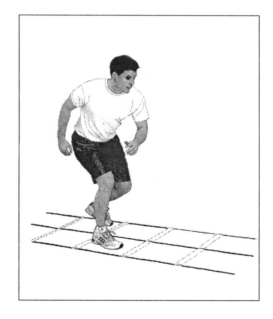

Drill: Backward In and Outs

Execution: Execute the same foot pattern as front in and outs, except this time move backwards from rung to rung until the end of the ladder. Repeat for the required number of repetitions. Some trainers suggest that front and back in and outs be alternated within the same drill.

Drill: Lateral In and Outs

Execution: Standing parallel to the first rung of an agility ladder, step in the first rung with your outside foot. Once your outside foot lands, immediately step in the same rung with your inside foot. After the inside foot lands, continue by stepping outside the ladder with your outside foot. Follow immediately by stepping outside the ladder with your inside foot. Proceed in the same pattern moving gradually to the end of the ladder, always concentrating on spending as little time as possible with your feet on the ground. Once the end of the ladder is reached, reverse course and repeat the pattern in the opposite direction. Continue for the required number of repetitions.

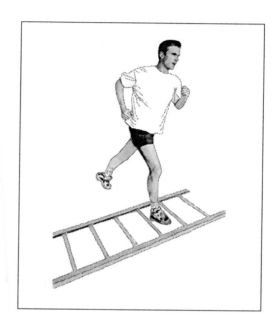

Specific Movement Pattern Drills

Drill: Side Shuffle

Execution: Begin in an athletic-ready stance (on the balls of your feet, knees comfortably flexed, feet at shoulder width, back taut, and head straight) and proceed to side shuffle (slide sideways without crossing your feet) back and forth over an eight-yard course for the required time or number of repetitions.

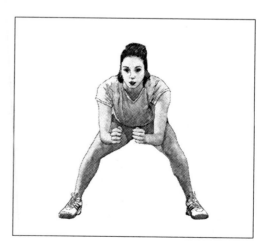

Drill: Three-Cone Short Shuttle

Execution: Place three cones in a triangular pattern spaced eight yards apart from each other. Begin in an athletic stance behind one of the cones. On "go," sprint to the cone on your left, touch it, and immediately reverse course and sprint back to the starting cone. From there, reestablish the athletic position briefly, and proceed by sprinting to the cone on your right, touch it, and immediately reverse course and sprint back to the starting cone. Repeat this pattern for two to six round trips.

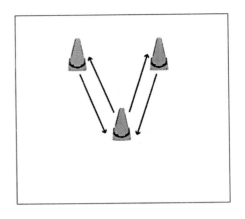

Drill: Sprint, Side Shuffle, Backpedal

Execution: Assume an athletic stance on an open field or court. On command, sprint eight yards straight ahead. Then, proceed to side shuffle five yards to your left. From there, immediately backpedal for eight yards. Repeat the pattern, but this time side shuffle to the right instead of the left. Complete two to six round trips.

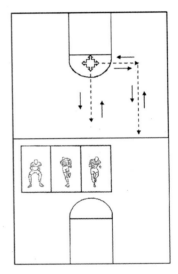

Drill: Mini-Cone Shuffle

Execution: Place a series of mini-cones or other low-lying barriers a foot or so apart. Using small side steps, shuffle over the cones/objects without crossing your feet, always concentrating on spending as little time as possible on the ground. When the end of the line is reached, reverse course and shuffle in the other direction. Repeat for the required time or number of repetitions.

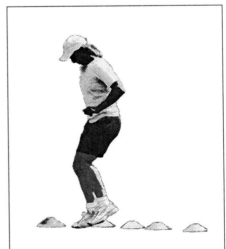

Drill: Lateral High Knees

Execution: Line up 12 to 14 barriers spaced three to four feet apart. The barriers can range in height from six to 18 inches, depending on the size and athletic ability of the youngster. Begin by stepping laterally with knees high and without crossing your feet over the barriers to the end of the line. After the last barrier is crossed, reverse course and repeat the pattern in the opposite direction. Continue for the required number of repetitions.

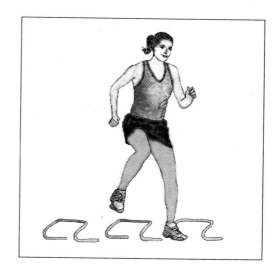

Drill: Vertical Half-Backs

Execution: Line up four lines of four cones each parallel to each other. The lines should measure approximately six to eight yards forward, and the space between each line will be about three to four feet, depending on the size of the young participant. Begin just behind the left line of cones. On "go," sprint to the top of the first line, change direction quickly, and

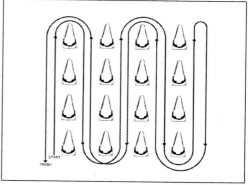

then backpedal as fast as possible between lines one and two. When the end of the line of cones is reached, change direction again and sprint between lines two and three. Follow the pattern to the end of the last line of cones. From there, reverse course and repeat the same pattern moving in the other direction. Continue for the required number of repetitions.

Drill: Horizontal Half-Backs

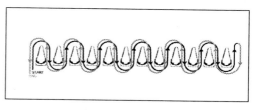

Execution: Line up 10 to 14 cones each approximately three feet apart. Begin by standing sideways just behind the first

cone. On "go," proceed to move quickly between each cone using forward, lateral, and back steps. Once the end of the line is reached, reverse course and repeat the pattern in the opposite direction. Continue for the required number of repetitions. For best results, short, choppy steps should be incorporated throughout.

Random Movement Pattern Drills

Drill: Side Shuffle on Command

Execution: Start as always in an athletic ready stance. Have a coach or training partner shout, "Move," and proceed to side shuffle to the left. When the coach/training partner shouts "Move" again, respond by changing direction quickly and side shuffling to the right. Continue for the required time.

Drill: Change Direction on Command

Execution: Assume an athletic stance. Position a coach or training partner facing you at approximately 15 feet away. Respond to commands of the coach/training partner to either side shuffle left or right, backpedal, or sprint straight ahead. Continue for the required time.

Drill: Colored Cone Wheel Response Drill

Execution: Arrange eight different colored cones in a star pattern equidistant at eight yards from a center cone (starting position). Assume an athletic stance just behind the center cone. Then, have a coach or training partner call out a color. Respond to the command by sprinting to the appropriate cone, touching it, and then sprinting back to the starting position. Reestablish an athletic stance and repeat. Continue for the required number of repetitions. Different movement patterns (such as side shuffles and backpedals) can be substituted for straight ahead sprints periodically for this drill.

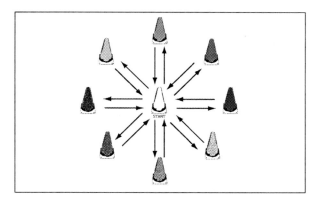

Drill: Bean Bag Toss and Catch

Execution: Stand facing a partner six to eight feet apart, each holding a small beanbag in one hand. (A tennis or squash ball can be used in lieu of the beanbag.) Proceed to side shuffle back and forth across a field or court while softly tossing the beanbags to each other in unison. The length of the course can range anywhere from eight to 15 yards, depending on the skill and conditioning of the participants. As youngsters become more proficient at the drill, encourage them to incorporate more difficult-to-handle throws (in front, behind, high, low, etc.). Continue for the required time or number of throws.

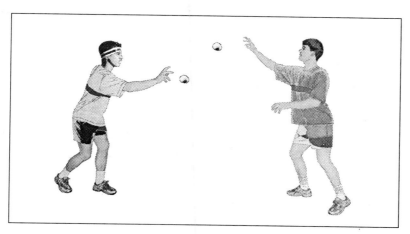

Drill: Reaction Belt Response Drill

Execution: To start, both youngsters will fasten a five foot long, Velcro reaction belt to their waists. One partner will then proceed, in no set pattern, to make a series of quick, unpredictable movements while the other partner attempts to follow as closely as possible. The object of the drill is to keep the belt on as long as possible without it breaking free, preferably for the duration of the drill. For best results, try to engage a partner who is quicker and more agile than you are.[1]

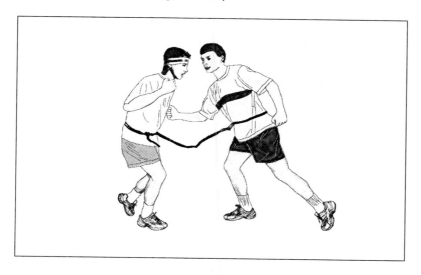

Drill: Reaction Ball Chase

Execution: Assume an athletic-ready stance facing a coach or training partner. Then, have the coach/training partner drop or toss a reaction ball (a small, ridged ball that bounces in unpredictable fashion). Proceed to chase the ball down, pick it up, and return it a fast as possible to the coach/training partner. Repeat for the required number of repetitions. To add a degree of competition to the drill, coaches/training partners should time each repetition.

Drill: Jog and Cut on Command

Execution: Delineate an approximately 30-yard long, 15-yard wide course using either lines or cones as markers. Begin by jogging slowly from the mid-point of the far end of the course while facing a coach/training partner situated at the top of the course. Respond to the coach/training partner's command to either cut "side left," "side right," "left front," "right front," "left back," or "right back." Side commands will entail sprinting laterally to the appropriate sideline and then sprinting back to the center of the course. Front and back commands will entail sprinting diagonally at a 45-degree angle either front or back to the appropriate sideline and then sprinting directly back to the center line. Once the athlete returns to the center of the course, he will continue his deliberate jog forward. It is important for this drill that the coach/training partner has a solid background in agility training. The jog and cut drill is usually executed for 20 to 30 seconds, but can be extended for conditioning purposes.

12

Plyometrics

Plyometrics, or "jump training" as it was originally called in Europe, is a form of explosiveness training that involves a series of jumps, hops, bounds, pushes, and medicine ball throws. It is designed to link speed with strength to produce power. This power is achieved by stretching or, in strength and conditioning vernacular, "loading" the muscles as fast as possible prior to a forceful contraction. Perhaps the best way to understand how plyometrics works is to think of muscles as rubber bands stretched to capacity then abruptly released, allowing the force and energy to move explosively in the opposite direction.

Plyometrics has numerous proponents throughout the youth sports community, along with its fair share of detractors. Advocates feel that proper and regular plyometric training greatly enhances a young athlete's ability to maneuver explosively during athletic competition. The cynics, on the other hand, are of the opinion that this high impact activity is just too dangerous for young, developing competitors, and is more likely to cause injury than it is to facilitate a higher vertical jump or a quicker first step.

While both camps offer articulate and persuasive arguments—not to mention numerous studies to back them up—there is a happy medium when it comes to youth plyometric training. The medium lies in the conscientious prescribing of age, physical maturity, and ability-appropriate plyometric workouts by coaches, trainers, and conditioning specialists. Simply put, some youngsters are better suited for basic plyometric exercises (i.e., broad jumps, tuck jumps, basic medicine ball throws), others for intermediate drills (i.e., barrier hops, power skips, lateral jumps) and a reasonably-sized minority for advanced movements (i.e., box jumps, plyometric push-ups, medicine ball squat jumps). As long as this protocol is adhered to, plyometrics can and should be a part of every young athlete's conditioning/sports improvement program.

Developing a Plyometric Program for Young Athletes

A number of factors should be taken into account when designing a plyometric program for youngsters, including the following.

Equipment

Although many plyometric drills can be executed without equipment, coaches, trainers, parents, and youngsters should be familiar with the following accessories.

Barriers. Barriers are incorporated in a variety of plyometric drills. They can range in height from six inches to as high as two feet, depending on the nature of the drill and the athletic ability of the youngster. The safest barriers are made of foam padding (recommended for Phase 1 children). The most widely used are plastic banana steps. Simple cones are also regularly utilized for plyometric training. Obviously, hard objects should never be used as a plyometric barrier.

Boxes. Boxes used for plyometrics should be sturdy, have semi-soft, non-slip landing surfaces, and range from one foot to over three feet in height. The top of the box (landing surface) should measure a minimum of 18 to 24 inches. Any less of a landing area would be dangerous. Because of the popularity of plyometrics in the sports conditioning community in recent years, specialized, height-adjustable plyometric boxes have been developed and are available for sale through most sporting goods outlets and fitness catalogs. However, homemade boxes work just as well, as long as they are built with the features described here.

Medicine balls. Medicine balls are incorporated in a variety of conditioning disciplines, some of which have been previously detailed in this book. For plyometric training purposes, they are used for executing a variety of different throws as well as squat jumps.

Weighted vests. The weighted vest is an outstanding tool for increasing explosiveness. Many athletes in jump-oriented sports such as volleyball and basketball routinely make use of this equipment in their plyometric training. Because the resistance is evenly distributed throughout the upper torso, plyometric drills performed while wearing a weighted vest are relatively safe. The vest weight to body weight ratio was discussed in the chapter on speed training (Chapter 10). The same parameters apply for plyometrics.

Training Surface

All plyometric training should be executed on soft surfaces. Rubberized running tracks, specially-made plyometric training pads, and low-cut grass are best. Wood flooring is acceptable, albeit somewhat more taxing on the joints than the other surfaces mentioned. Engaging in plyometrics on hard surfaces, such as pavement or on uneven terrain, should be avoided. No exceptions.

Footwear

Because the large majority of plyometric exercises are of the high-impact variety, it is essential that youngsters wear proper training shoes during plyometric workouts. Basketball/cross-training sneakers are suggested. This type of footwear provides lateral support, is sufficiently cushioned, and has non-slip soles; all required features for safe plyometric training. Running or jogging shoes lack lateral stability and leave young athletes susceptible to twisted knees and ankles; thus they are discouraged for plyometric workouts. Unless working out in the sand, plyometrics should never be performed barefoot.

Program Length

The length of a young athlete's plyometric program will depend on a host of variables including (but not limited to) sport(s), age, physical maturity, athletic ability, strength and conditioning level, and body type. Most programs will last between 12 to 16 off-season weeks. Engaging in regular plyometric training while participating in a sports season, especially if the sport is explosively oriented (football, basketball, volleyball, lacrosse, etc.), is too much for most youngsters to tolerate from a physical standpoint and will often lead to overtraining and injury.

Workouts Per Week

Plyometric workouts, because of their demanding nature, should be accomplished no more than two times per week. The individual sessions will always be separated by a minimum of 48 to 72 hours.

Sets and Repetitions

As with strength training, the number of sets and repetitions per workout will vary with a young athlete's needs and ability. Typically, a total of 100 foot contacts (repetitions) should occur for Phase 1 children, 150 foot contacts for Phase 2 youngsters, and up to 200 foot contacts for Phase 3 athletes. For best results (and to keep plyometric training as interesting as possible), the repetitions should be spread among three to four or more different drills. The repetition range will be between 6 and 15 per set.

Rest Between Sets

The level of intensity at which the young athlete is training will determine the rest between sets of plyometric exercises. For warm-up and low-intensity sets, one-minute rest intervals should be sufficient. High intensity efforts will require up to three minutes of rest before beginning the next set.

Physical Preparation

Proper physical preparation is, without question, the most important factor to successful, injury-free youth plyometric training. Engaging in these demanding workouts without a solid strength and conditioning base is a recipe for failure, not to mention frustration and injury.

Young athletes must have a minimum of 10 to 12 weeks of consistent strength training behind them prior to embarking on a plyometric program. Lower-body strength is most important, as jumping and landing are the key components of plyometrics. Solid cardiovascular conditioning and a reasonable degree of flexibility are also prerequisites for engaging in plyometric workouts.

Proper Execution

Performing plyometric drills correctly is essential to safe and effective workouts. The high impact and somewhat complicated nature of the discipline will require that young athletes pay close attention to execution or risk injury. For best results, coaches and trainers should require that young athletes perform their first few plyometric sessions at half speed, focusing on technique and form, rather than velocity and intensity. It is also advisable that youth coaches enlist an experienced sports training specialist for a plyometrics demonstration prior to program commencement.

Progression

Once proper technique is mastered, youngsters of all phases should aspire to progress from simpler plyometric movements to the more advanced variety. Intensity should be ramped up as well. Progression (as is the case in all training disciplines) is the name of the game in plyometrics.

Effort and Intensity

Plyometric drills are designed to be performed at a high level of intensity. Once warm-up sets are concluded, it is essential that every movement in a young athlete's plyometric workout be executed with all-out effort.

Final Word: Don't Overdo It

Just to re-emphasize, while performance-enhancing for young athletes, plyometrics is an extremely demanding form of physical conditioning—one that if overdone can cause body breakdown for even the most physically gifted of youngsters. As such, coaches and trainers should remain reasonably conservative when prescribing plyometric workout programs to the young athletes under their guidance.

Plyometric Drills

A variety of plyometric drills are detailed in the following sections. The skill levels range from simple to advanced. While the exercises provided are certainly more than sufficient to structure a challenging plyometric program for young athletes, they are only a small slice of the plyometric-drill pie. Potentially, hundreds of plyometric drills are available to young athletes. As such, youngsters are encouraged, with the appropriate guidance from their coaches and trainers, to include additional drills in their programs, or even develop their own as their individual training objectives dictate.

Drill: Jump and Reach

Execution: Assume an erect and balanced stance with your head up and eyes fixed straight ahead. Proceed by bending quickly into jumping position (thighs approximately three-quarters to parallel) and instantaneously explode upward, reaching up with one hand as high as possible. Repeat alternating reaching hands for the required number of repetitions.

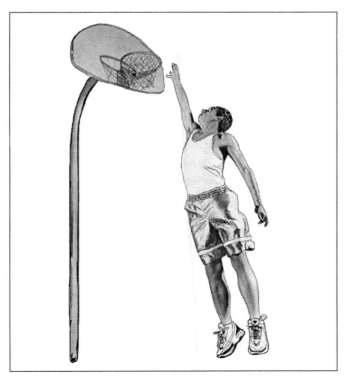

Drill: Double-Leg Tuck Jump

Execution: Assume an erect and balanced stance with your head up, eyes fixed straight ahead, and arms positioned straight out in front of you. Continue by bending quickly to the jumping position and immediately spring straight up as high as you can, while concurrently pulling your knees up to your chest. Repeat for the required number of repetitions.

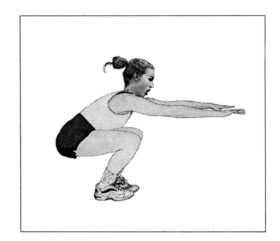

Drill: Broad Jump

Execution: With your feet shoulder-width apart, knees flexed, and arms at your sides, broad jump as high and as far forward as you can. During the airborne phase of the drill, your upper body should be in a straight line. Repeat for the required number of repetitions.

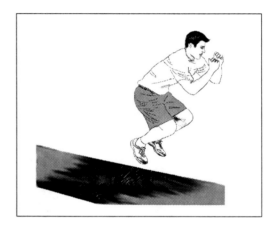

Drill: Power Skips

Execution: Starting in a slow jog, gradually pick up speed, exaggerating your arm swing and knee lift. Your upper leg of the driving knee should be slightly above parallel to the running surface. The objective is to cover as much ground as possible during the airborne phase of the drill.

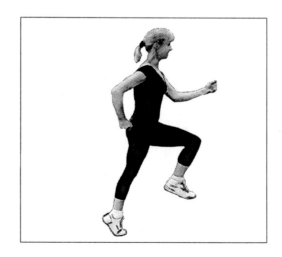

Drill: Medicine Ball Shoulder Toss

Execution: Standing erect, take hold of an appropriately-weighted medicine ball and position it directly overhead with your elbows bent so that they are approximately at ear height. Proceed to bend at the knees to just short of jumping position and immediately reverse direction, straightening your legs and concurrently releasing the ball straight up as high as possible. During the catch phase of the drill, try to keep your hands above your head (which keeps the tension on the shoulders). Continue for the required number of repetitions.

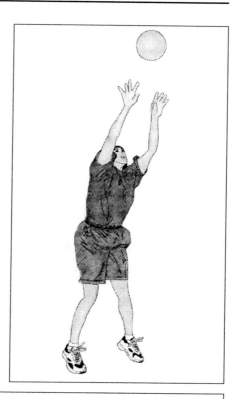

Drill: Backward Medicine Ball Toss

Execution: Stand with your knees bent and your feet slightly wider than shoulder width and pick up an appropriately-weighted medicine ball from the floor. Proceed to swing the ball between your legs and, as your forearms come just short of your thighs, reverse course and throw the ball powerfully over your head as far as possible. Repeat for the required number of repetitions.

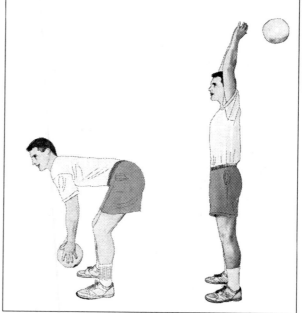

Drill: Medicine Ball Side Wall Toss

Execution: Standing perpendicular to a wall three to five feet away with your knees slightly flexed, grab hold of an appropriately-weighted medicine ball and position it near your far hip. Proceed to swing the ball powerfully across your body and release it toward the wall at waist height. Catch the rebound, and continue in rapid-fire fashion for the required number of repetitions. Reverse standing position and repeat.

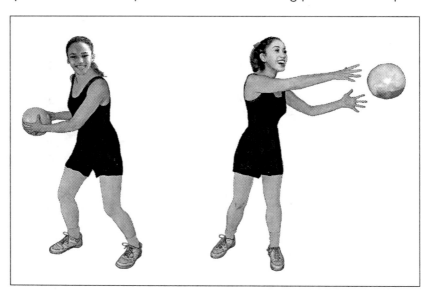

Drill: Lateral Barrier Jumps

Execution: Place a barrier of appropriate height on the ground and stand sideways to it in the athletic position. Proceed to jump laterally back and forth over the barrier for the required number of repetitions.

Drill: Over and Backs

Execution: Stand in the athletic position facing a barrier of appropriate height. Proceed to jump over it. Then, immediately upon landing, reverse course and jump backwards over the barrier to the starting position. Repeat back and forth for the required number of repetitions.

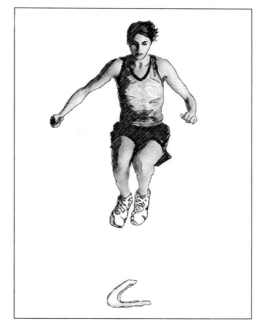

Drill: Multiple Front Barrier Jumps

Execution: Line up 10 to 14 appropriately-sized barriers, spaced approximately three feet apart. Begin in the athletic position facing the line, and proceed to jump over each barrier until the end of the line. Turn 180 degrees and repeat the pattern. Continue for the required number of round trips.

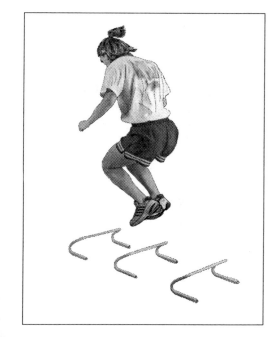

Drill: Multiple Lateral Barrier Jumps

Execution: Line up two to four appropriately-sized barriers, spaced approximately three feet apart. Begin in the athletic position sideways to the line, and proceed to jump laterally over each barrier. After the last barrier is cleared, shift your weight to the outside leg and repeat in the opposite direction. Continue for the required number of round trips.

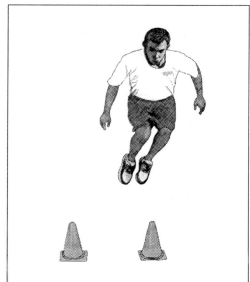

Drill: Staggered Barrier Jumps

Execution: Position 12 barriers of appropriate height in a staggered pattern three to four feet apart. From the athletic position, proceed to jump diagonally over each barrier. When the last barrier is cleared, turn 180 degrees and repeat the pattern. Continue for the require number of round trips.

Drill: Box Push-Offs

Execution: Stand with one foot placed on an appropriately sized box, with your other foot planted firmly on the ground. With the raised knee slightly flexed, push off powerfully and jump straight up as high as possible. Reverse your legs in the air and land under control with your opposite leg on the box. Your arms will swing as if running in place. Repeat in rapid fashion for the duration of the drill.

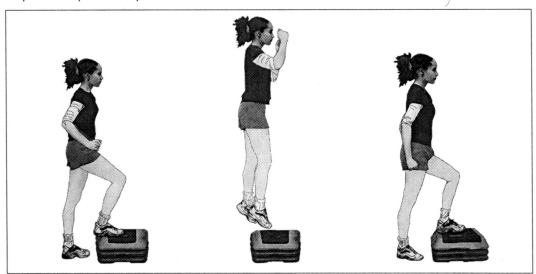

Drill: Front Box Jumps

Execution: Stand in the athletic position facing an appropriately-sized box. Proceed to jump up on to the box, landing under control on both feet. Hop down quickly, and upon touching the ground, immediately jump back up. Repeat for the required number of repetitions.

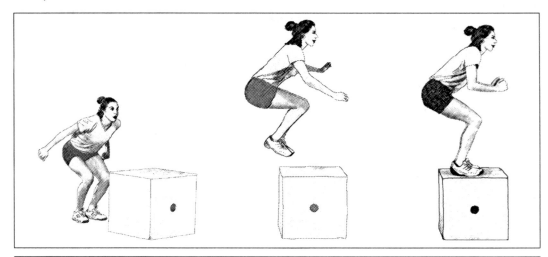

Drill: Lateral Box Jumps

Execution: Stand sideways to an appropriately-sized box in the athletic position. Begin by jumping laterally up on to the box, landing under control on both feet. Hop down quickly and, upon touching the ground, immediately jump back up. Repeat for the required number of repetitions. Alternate sides each set.

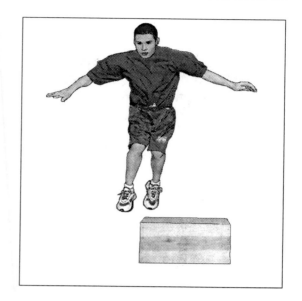

Drill: Front Box Jump with Step Down

Execution: Stand facing an appropriately-sized box in the athletic position. Jump on to the box, landing under control on two feet. Pause briefly, then step down off the box, drop to the floor, and immediately spring into the air as high as possible (one repetition). Repeat for the required number of repetitions.

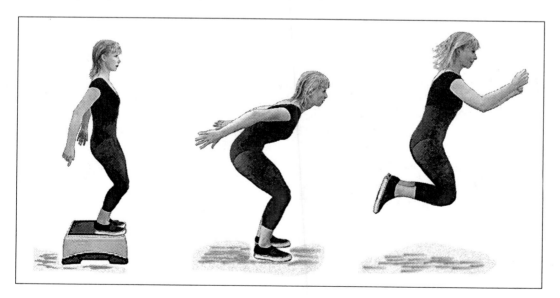

Drill: Multiple Box Jumps

Execution: Line up three to five one-foot high boxes, spaced three to five feet apart. Face the line in the athletic position, and proceed to jump on and off each box in succession until the end of the row. Walk back deliberately to the starting position and repeat. Continue for the required number of repetitions.

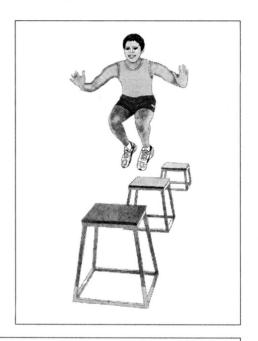

Drill: Medicine Ball Squat Jump

Execution: Begin by assuming a shoulder-width stance with your feet pointed slightly outward. Take hold of an appropriately-weighted medicine ball and place it comfortably behind your neck. Proceed to squat down until your upper legs are approximately parallel to the floor and then explode upward as high as possible. The ball should stay in contact with your neck and shoulders throughout the drill. Repeat for the required number of repetitions. A weighted vest can be incorporated in lieu of a medicine ball for this drill.

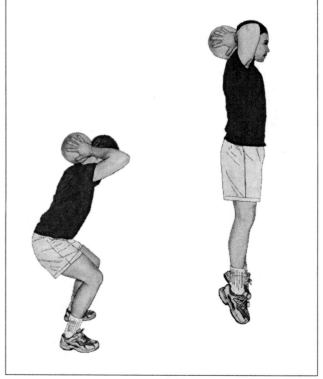

Drill: Plyometric Push-Up

Execution: With your feet raised approximately six inches, assume a conventional push-up position. Begin by pushing up explosively, allowing your hands to leave the ground. When your hands return to the ground, catch yourself, and immediately explode upward for another repetition. Repeat for the required number of repetitions.

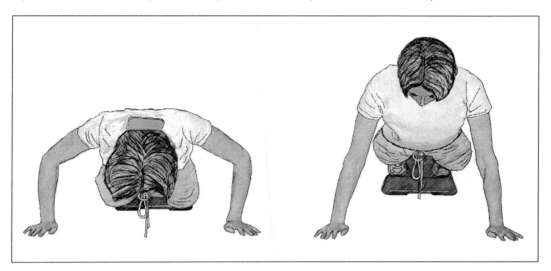

13

Cross Training

Cross training, as the name suggests, entails incorporating a variety of different exercise modalities into a workout or workout program. This technique provides numerous athletic and performance benefits, helps to prevent overuse injuries caused by repetitive activity, and perhaps most importantly for young athletes, keeps training sessions fresh, interesting, and creative. The following are a number of cross training options appropriate for young athletes.

Jumping Rope

Jumping rope has been a fitness staple for generations. Originally popular in the boxing world because of its overall conditioning and footwork benefits, rope jumping is perhaps the one exercise method used regularly in virtually every sport from basketball to figure skating. Depending on how they're implemented, jump-rope workouts can enhance numerous aspects of athletic performance—including aerobic and anaerobic conditioning, balance, quickness/agility, strength, power/explosiveness, coordination, and speed. Needless to say, all young athletes should own a jump rope.

Basics of Safe and Effective Jump Rope Workouts

Jump rope length. A jump rope should be long enough to reach armpit to armpit, while passing under both shoulder width spread feet.

Types of jump ropes. The three basic types of jump ropes are: light-handled, heavy-handled, and heavy-corded. Each has it own unique performance-enhancing features.

A light-handled rope is best for promoting hand speed, foot quickness, and general coordination. It is also great tool for improving aerobic conditioning, as the rope's easy-turning feature allows athletes to jump for extended periods of time without tiring. Phase 1 youngsters will incorporate this type of rope exclusively in their rope-jumping workouts.

Jumping with a heavy-handled rope will greatly improve hand, wrist, and forearm strength, along with providing those youngsters who are ready (late Phase 2 and Phase 3 athletes) a terrific lactic acid system workout.

Exercising with a heavy-corded rope is appropriate for Phase 3 athletes only. It provides an extremely intense workout, one that stimulates the ATP-PC and lactic acid systems of the anaerobic metabolism and strengthens the muscles of the upper body (especially the shoulders) to a high degree.

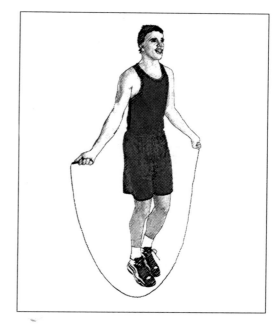

Turning the jump rope. Turning a jump rope is a fairly simple process. It entails turning the hands and wrists in a natural forward circle. The upper arms should be held close to the torso, and the forearms should be pointed downward at an approximately 45-degree angle during execution.

Where to jump. It is best that youngsters conduct their rope jumping workouts on semi-soft surfaces—wood flooring, rubberized running tracks, and artificial turf are all ideal. Specially-designed jump rope mats are also available through a variety of fitness catalogs and sporting goods stores. Be aware, however, that these floor coverings provide a "quick rebound" effect that requires the athlete to have some degree of rope jumping expertise. As such, Phase 1 youngsters and/or older, beginning rope jumpers should garner some rope jumping experience before incorporating this equipment. Hard surfaces such as concrete or asphalt should be avoided when jumping rope, as should uneven terrain.

Jumping patterns. Although virtually hundreds of jumping patterns are available to choose from when jumping rope, the following three basic methods should be enough for youngsters to enjoy productive, conditioning-promoting workouts:
- Two-foot jump: The youngster jumps once each rope turn, with both feet hitting the ground simultaneously. The feet should be slightly closer than shoulder-width when executing this jumping pattern.

- Alternate foot jump: The youngster jumps once each rope turn, alternating landings between his left and right foot. Jumping in this manner resembles running in place.
- Skip jump: The youngster jumps once each rope turn, alternating landings in no set sequence between left foot, right foot, and both feet simultaneously.

Once these techniques are mastered, youngsters are encouraged to learn and perfect more complicated jumping patterns, especially if jumping rope becomes a large part of their workout regimen.

Station Training

Station training consists of a series of exercise posts in which athletes perform a different conditioning activity at each stop. For instance, one station may entail jumping rope, another body weight squats, and the next push-ups or bench dips. The number of stations, the time spent exercising within each station, and the total station circuits accomplished will depend on the age, experience, and conditioning level of the youngster involved.

Diversity is an important factor in successful station workouts. Mixing up exercise options will help youngsters develop balanced athletic ability and make the training session more interesting as well. All components of conditioning—from strength to endurance—should be represented in these workouts, if possible.

Older, more physically-mature athletes (late Phase 2 and Phase 3 youngsters) should aspire to move from station to station fairly quickly, challenging themselves as much as possible from a conditioning standpoint. Younger children (Phase 1 and early Phase 2 youngsters) will be more deliberate within the circuit and are encouraged to work hard but at their own pace. For obvious reasons, station training lends itself to group workouts. Table 13-1 provides an example of a station workout.

| Station #1: Rope jumping |
| Station #2: Push-ups |
| Station #3: Ball twists |
| Station #4: Body weight squats |
| Station #5: Inverted chin-ups |
| Station #6: Lateral barrier hops |

Table 13-1. Sample station training workout

Chase the Rabbit Relay

Youngsters have participated in and enjoyed relay races for generations. Not only have relays proved to be a great form of exercise, one that increases both speed and stamina, but they encourage teamwork and a sense of camaraderie between youngsters as well. And, of course, they are extremely fun for all involved—including supervisors and coaches.

The "chase the rabbit" relay race was developed by a group of enterprising young baseball coaches who wanted to improve the speed and technical base-running ability of their players in a fun and semi-competitive manner. Here's how it works. Four bases are set up equidistant from each other, as they would be on a baseball or softball diamond. (The size of the diamond will depend on available space and the age and athletic ability of the youngsters participating.) The group of young athletes will then be split up into two equal sized teams, with one team lined up single file behind the base representing home plate and the other team doing the same behind second base. On "go," the first two youngsters in each line will sprint counter-clockwise around the entire diamond, touching each base as they go. Once the starting/finishing base (either home or second) is reached, the next athlete in line will take off at full-speed and repeat the process. The drill ends when a member of one team overtakes or touches a member of the other team.

To avoid collision and to make sure that the drill is run properly, youngsters in line should always remain a few feet behind their starting base until their teammate crosses it. To ensure that this happens, it is suggested that an adult supervisor be stationed at both starting/finishing bases. Because the "chase the rabbit" relay tends to last a reasonably long time until a winner emerges, a minimum of eight youngsters per team is recommended. This type of training, while appropriate for all age groups, is most popular with younger children.

Speed Play

Speed play, or "fartlek training" as it was called when it originated decades ago in Sweden, involves running at different speeds for arbitrary intervals of time or distance. The distance and pace chosen are totally up to the runner or the coach leading the drill. Many conditioning experts feel that speed play is tailor-made for competitive athletes because it creates an atmosphere of non-planned speed changes similar to what occurs in most sports. The technique also provides substantial aerobic and anaerobic conditioning benefits in the same workout.

Notwithstanding the conditioning benefits, speed play is especially appealing to youngsters for another reason: it's fun. Most young athletes find even-paced running or jogging somewhat boring; on the other hand, traversing a challenging course at various speeds is exhilarating and concentration inducing, which allows time, perceptually at least, to pass more quickly—an important factor during a grueling conditioning run

Running paths with soft surfaces and a reasonable compliment of hills, turns, and flat straight-aways are ideal for speed play. However, these workouts can be just as easily accomplished running on a track, around a perimeter of a football or soccer field, or though a low-trafficked residential neighborhood. Speed play, depending on the goals and capabilities of the youngster, can range from 15 minutes to over an hour. Table 13-2 illustrates an example of a speed play training session.

Jog: 5 minutes > **Stride:** 3 minutes > **Jog:** 2 minutes > **Sprint:** 90 seconds >
Jog: 1 minute > **Stride:** 2 minutes > **Sprint:** 1 minute > **Jog:** 3 minutes >
Sprint: 30 seconds > **Stride:** 2 minutes > **Jog:** 2 minutes > **Sprint:** 1 minute >
Stride: 1 minute > **Jog:** 2 minutes > **Sprint:** 90 seconds > **Jog:** 1 minute >
Sprint: 30 seconds > **Jog:** 1 minute

Table 13-2. Sample fartlek training session

Sand Workouts

Sand workouts are a great addition to any young athlete's training regime. They produce significant improvements in cardiovascular fitness, lower-body strength, and athleticism; are extremely safe and easy on the joints, bones, and muscles; and provide an enjoyable and refreshing change of pace—especially for those youngsters who take the majority of their conditioning workouts indoors.

All types of movement-oriented training are appropriate for the sand. Some of the most popular and effective sand drills include shuttle runs (runs that entail a variety of movement patterns, such as straight ahead sprints, side shuffles, and backpedals), explosive plyometric exercises, and random pattern agility training. Youngsters should feel free to experiment with different exercises on the sand as they would anywhere else.

A scenic, even landscaped beach is the ideal setting for sand workouts. If this backdrop is not available, check local high schools and colleges, as many now feature man-made sand pits specifically designed for athletic training. If all else fails, a simple sand box or long jump pit will suffice.

Before beginning each and every sand-training session, especially if it's taking place on a public beach, check the terrain carefully for sharp objects such as cracked seashells, jagged edged rocks, and broken glass. Sand workouts can be executed barefoot or while wearing a variety of training footwear.

Boxing Training

Boxers are universally recognized as among the best-conditioned athletes in the world. Because of the grueling nature of their sport, fighters must train their bodies comprehensively and rigorously, leaving no stone unturned from a fitness standpoint. Unlike most athletes, boxers who come to competition out of shape risk not only losing, but exposing themselves to serious injury as well.

Young athletes of all ages can benefit greatly by incorporating boxing workouts into their year-round conditioning programs. The sessions themselves include virtually all facets of physical conditioning and athletic enhancement training. For example, pounding away on the heavy bag strengthens the hands, wrists, arms, upper back and shoulders, while at the same time giving the bodies anaerobic system all it can handle. Speed bag work enhances hand-eye coordination and increases hand speed. Jumping rope promotes foot quickness, coordination, and endurance. A variety of abdominal and medicine ball exercises will increase power in the all-important core of the body. In-ring drills with a trainer will help to develop balance, footwork, and timing. And above all, engaging in regular boxing workouts engenders discipline and toughness—both obviously crucial to sports success.

All boxing workouts for young athletes will be supervised by an experienced boxing trainer, preferably one who has competed regularly in the squared circle. Under no circumstances should youngsters go it alone in the boxing gym. The precise training methods involved require expert appraisal throughout the workout. While many commercial health and fitness clubs now offer boxing classes, the best way to learn the "sweet science" is at an old-fashion boxing gym. These facilities supply the best trainers, include the proper boxing equipment, and provide an atmosphere most conducive to productive boxing workouts. Table 13-3 presents a sample boxing workout.

1 round shadow boxing (warm-up)	2 rounds in-ring footwork drills
2 rounds rope skipping	2 rounds rope skipping
3 rounds heavy bag work	2 rounds abdominal training
2 rounds speed bag work	1 round shadow boxing (cool-down)

▶ The workout is based on three-minute rounds and one-minute rest intervals between rounds.

Table 13-3. A sample boxing workout

Obstacle Course

Obstacle course races have been around for decades. They can regularly be seen taking place during gym classes, in schoolyards, and at family picnics throughout the country and the world. The obstacle course was even the final and most important (not to mention the most challenging) event in the popular Superstars competition where world-class competitors from a variety of sports vied on national television for the title of best all-round athlete.

Perhaps the best feature of working through an obstacle course—other than the fun of it—is that engages practically all the components of strength, conditioning, and athleticism. Quickness, agility, balance, strength, speed, explosiveness, cardiovascular fitness—you name it and traversing a challenging obstacle course requires it. In many ways, obstacle courses provide the ultimate circuit training vehicle, demanding that young athletes move as fast as possible from one exercise discipline to another without hesitation or rest.

Obstacle course training is appropriate for all phases of athletic development. However, the length and difficultly of the course will depend on the age and physical capabilities of the youngsters involved. Program directors and trainers are encouraged to be creative in designing obstacle courses, making them diverse, challenging, and fun. Safety, of course, is also a priority when setting up an obstacle course. Race competition should be tempered for Phase 1 children, with the focus being on proper negotiation of the course as opposed to speed. Older youngsters can and are encouraged to compete wholeheartedly in obstacle course races. When a large group (eight and up) of youngsters are involved, incorporating a relay race format is suggested. Table 13-4 provides a sample obstacle course workout.

• Start	• Sprint five yards
• Sprint five yards	• Monkey bar hand-over-hand traverse (six to eight rungs)
• Blocking sled push (seven yards)	• Under barrier
• Sprint 10 yards	• Over low hurdle
• Long jump	• Sprint eight yards
• High knee tire run (four to six sets of tires)	• Wall scale (height depends on age and athletic ability of youngster)
• Sprint 10 yards	• Sprint 12 yards
• High jump	• Finish

Table 13-4. Sample obstacle course

Medicine Ball Slides

The ability to move laterally is of paramount importance in a variety of sports. Just a few examples when this skill comes into play include fielding a ground ball in baseball or softball, playing defense in basketball and soccer, and sliding into position to return a hot tennis serve.

A great drill for developing lateral movement is medicine ball slides. The action combines a controlled side-to-side motion with a resistance component (the ball), which if performed regularly leads to improvements in balance, overall body strength, and lateral speed. General footwork will be enhanced as well.

Execution is fairly simple (simple, not easy). Begin by holding an appropriately-weighted medicine ball (some Phase 1 children may want to start with a basketball or volleyball) at chest height with arms extended approximately 80 percent. The ball will be held in this position for the duration of the drill. Proceed by sliding laterally without crossing the feet in one direction for 10 to 15 yards. Then, reverse course and slide back in the same fashion to the starting point. How many times a youngster covers the course will depend on their level of strength and conditioning.

To add a degree of difficulty and reality to the drill, young athletes can slide at various angles, giving or gaining ground gradually on each length. This technique will better simulate live sports action. For variety, and to incorporate an element of hand-eye coordination, medicine ball slides can also be executed with two youngsters passing the ball back and forth over the duration of the course (see illustration). Finally, advanced young athletes (Phase 3) are encouraged to combine medicine ball slides with other conditioning/athletic enhancement disciplines. For example, have youngsters execute a 20- to 30-second set of lateral barrier hops, immediately followed by two round-trips of medicine ball slides, and ending with a 12-yard backpedal and a 12-yard sprint.

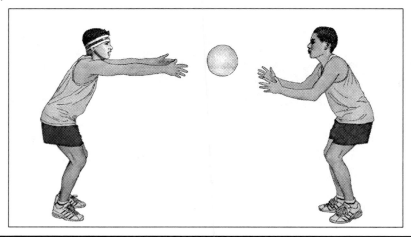

Wall Climbing

The sport of rock climbing has become increasingly popular in recent years. The activity bridges the gap between the outdoor and extreme sport communities, thus attracting a large cross-section of hardy and risk-tolerant athletes.

Rock climbing's popularity has also led many fitness gyms and health clubs to add state-of-the-art climbing walls. These structures allow individuals to basically simulate outdoor climbing in a controlled and safe environment.

Along with being fun, safe, mentally challenging, and group-friendly, wall climbing provides young athletes a fantastic workout—especially for those areas of the body that are frequently neglected in youth strength programs, such as the fingers, hands, wrists, forearms, and upper back. Regular work on the climbing wall also contributes to improving cardiovascular fitness as well

It is imperative that an experienced instructor be on hand for all climbing sessions. These individuals will teach and demonstrate proper climbing technique, along with ensuring that safety equipment is correctly secured to each participating youngster. Most of these climbing facilities employ competent instructors. However, it is still suggested that adults chaperoning youngsters (coaches, trainers, parents, etc.) interview potential instructors prior to climbing sessions so as to become comfortable with their skills and qualifications.

Youngsters are discouraged from racing each other up and down the wall during climbing sessions and horseplay is absolutely forbidden. These activities can be dangerous and they take away form the goal of the effort, which is to garner an effective and fun conditioning-promoting workout. Youngsters who are afraid of heights or are generally uncomfortable on a climbing wall should feel free to skip this cross training option.

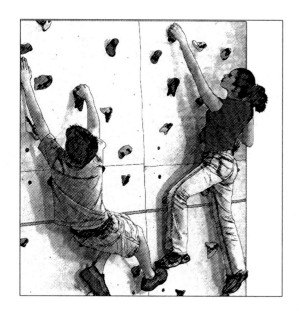